MW00627341

Quick Reference for the Lactation Professional

Judith Lauwers BA, IBCLC

Education Coordinator

International Lactation Consultant Association

Chalfont, Pennsylvania

JONES AND BARTLETT PUBLISHERS

Sudbury, Massachusetts

BOSTON   TORONTO   LONDON   SINGAPORE

World Headquarters

Jones and Bartlett Publishers
40 Tall Pine Drive
Sudbury, MA 01776
978-443-5000
info@jbpub.com
www.jbpub.com

Jones and Bartlett Publishers
Canada
6339 Ormindale Way
Mississauga, Ontario L5V 1J2
CANADA

Jones and Bartlett Publishers
International
Barb House, Barb Mews
London W6 7PA
UK

Jones and Bartlett's books and products are available through most bookstores and online booksellers. To contact Jones and Bartlett Publishers directly, call 800-832-0034, fax 978-443-8000, or visit our website, www.jbpub.com.

Substantial discounts on bulk quantities of Jones and Bartlett's publications are available to corporations, professional associations, and other qualified organizations. For details and specific discount information, contact the special sales department at Jones and Bartlett via the above contact information or send an email to specialsales@jbpub.com.

The authors, editor, and publisher have made every effort to provide accurate information. However, they are not responsible for errors, omissions, or for any outcomes related to the use of the contents of this book and take no responsibility for the use of the products and procedures described. Treatments and side effects described in this book may not be applicable to all people; likewise, some people may require a dose or experience a side effect that is not described herein. Drugs and medical devices are discussed that may have limited availability controlled by the Food and Drug Administration (FDA) for use only in a research study or clinical trial. Research, clinical practice, and government regulations often change the accepted standard in this field. When consideration is being given to use of any drug in the clinical setting, the health care provider or reader is responsible for determining FDA status of the drug, reading the package insert, and reviewing prescribing information for the most up-to-date recommendations on dose, precautions, and contraindications, and determining the appropriate usage for the product. This is especially important in the case of drugs that are new or seldom used.

Library of Congress Cataloging-in-Publication Data
Lauwers, Judith, 1949-
  Quick reference for the lactation professional / Judith Lauwers.
    p. ; cm.
  Includes bibliographical references and index.
  ISBN-13: 978-0-7637-5014-5 (alk. paper)
  ISBN-10: 0-7637-5014-X (alk. paper)
  1. Lactation consultants--Handbooks, manuals, etc. I. Title.
  [DNLM: 1. Breast Feeding--Handbooks. 2. Counseling--methods--Handbooks. 3. Lactation--Handbooks. 4. Patient Education as Topic--methods--Handbooks. WS 39 L391q 2008]
  RJ216.L355 2008
  649'.33--dc22
                            20070486226048

Production Credits
Executive Editor: Kevin Sullivan
Aquisitions Editor: Emily Ekle
Aquisitions Editor: Amy Sibley
Editorial Assistant: Patricia Donnelly
Production Director: Amy Rose
Associate Production Editor: Amanda Clerkin
Associate Marketing Manager: Rebecca Wasley

Manufacturing and Inventory Control Supervisor:
  Amy Bacus
Composition: Shawn Girsberger
Cover Design: Kate Ternullo
Cover Image: © Daniela Illing/ShutterStock, Inc.
Printing and Binding: Malloy, Inc.
Cover Printing: Malloy, Inc.

6048

Printed in the United States of America
13 12 11 10 09   10 9 8 7 6 5 4 3

Contents

Introduction

This *Quick Reference for the Lactation Professional* serves a dual purpose. First, it provides a convenient quick reference for clinicians working with mothers and babies. Second, it is an invaluable tool for educators, students, and interns with tutorials at the end of each chapter that test breastfeeding knowledge and application of theory to practice. Chapter content is based on material in the fourth edition of *Counseling the Nursing Mother: A Lactation Consultant's Guide*. The reader may refer to that text for references to support the information and recommendations in this guide.

Special Features at the End of Each Chapter

- Key clinical management strategies from *Clinical Guidelines for the Establishment of Exclusive Breastfeeding* relevant to the chapter topics
- Key clinical competencies from *Clinical Competencies for IBCLC Practice* relevant to the chapter topics—convenient for checking off competencies as they are completed
- Tutorial that includes short answer questions and counseling scenarios to test
- Comprehension and application of information to clinical practice

The Tutorials Can Be Used By:

- Educators who wish to assess students and interns as they prepare for the lactation profession
- Students and interns who want to track their learning of clinical management strategies and clinical competencies
- Candidates for the certification exam
- Those starting out in practice or updating their clinical skills and knowledge

Acknowledgments

I wish to express my gratitude to Karen Strube and Anna Swisher for their insights while reviewing chapters during the preparation of the manuscript. Thank you to innumerable colleagues who provide inspiration as I continue along my journey of lifelong learning. You know who you are! Thank you as well to the Jones and Bartlett staff for their guidance throughout the publication process.

Thank you to my husband, Dave, for his continuing support and patience. Thank you to my daughters-in-law Jennifer and Heather for providing inspiration as I delight in their parenting of my breastfed grandchildren Molly, Juliette, and Matthew. And thank you to my sons, Michael and Christopher, for marrying such nurturing women and for being remarkable fathers!

Judith Lauwers, BA, IBCLC
Education Coordinator, International Lactation Consultant Association
Lactation Consultant, Doylestown Hospital, Doylestown, Pennsylvania

CHAPTER 1

Insights into Mothers and Families

In This Chapter

Psychology and Motivation

Perception and Attitude

- Attributing causes for past events influences expectations of the future.
- What we *expect* to see influences what we *do* see.
- Needs, motives, attitudes, and reactions can motivate behavior change.
- Self-image influences actions.
- Attitudes, beliefs and values play roles in societal change.
- Social situations influence our thoughts, self-perception, and impressions of others.
- First impressions tend to be lasting.
- People can be stimulated below their level of conscious awareness.
- Attitude formation is linked to information, experience and influence of family and friends.
- Individuals are not always ready or willing to process a great deal of information.
- Needs and goals change in response to conditions, environment, experiences, and interactions.
- Lack of confidence, negative messages, and misconceptions about normal infant behavior and breastfeeding patterns can cause mothers to perceive insufficient milk production.

Behavior and Decision Making

- Roles we play in society determine our expectations and behavior.

    - Most behavior results from deliberation, judgment, beliefs, and expectations.
    - Unconscious needs or drives are at the heart of motivation and personality.
    - Central beliefs and values are resistant to change.
    - The family passes along basic cultural beliefs, values, and customs.

- Motivation, perception, learning, personality, and attitudes influence decision making.

    - Your personality affects your rapport with mothers.
    - Educated consumers respond to factual appeals.
    - Less educated consumers react to emotional appeals.
    - Highly involved individuals are likely to evaluate pros and cons in a message.
    - Humor increases acceptance and persuasiveness.
    - Building one influence upon another influence increases compliance.
    - Product, price, place, and promotion determine behavior change.

Empowerment

- Omitting information does not contribute to a trusting relationship.

    - Noncommittal messages compromise self-confidence and create doubt about decisions.
    - Appropriate guilt serves as motivation to change behavior.

- Mothers who exercise legitimate control feel more independent, self-reliant, and confident.

    - Positive self-image and confidence in parenting lead to positive attachments.
    - Taking control over their health needs empowers women to gain mastery over their lives.

- Outreach counseling and emotional support contribute to mothers reaching their goals.

ADVICE TO CLINICIANS
BE EMPOWERING

- ▶ Avoid making assumptions about mothers' motivations and goals.
- ▶ Expect that mothers will breastfeed unless they tell you otherwise.
- ▶ Avoid jumping to conclusions before examining all relevant information.
- ▶ Send a clear, positive message about the superiority of breastfeeding.

- Support groups educate women about options and help them make informed choices.
- Participating in a support group increases satisfaction and self-confidence.
- Mutual sharing and observing mothers breastfeed their babies enhances breastfeeding and parenting.

Family Dynamics
Becoming a Mother

- Mothers have a range of normal postpartum reactions.

  - They may feel isolated and lonely from the loss of adult contact.
  - They may feel a loss of control and inexperience in caring for a baby.
  - They may be anxious because of a fussy, high-need baby.

- **Baby blues** appear around the third day postpartum.

  - Bouts of tearfulness and sadness mingle with happiness and excitement.
  - Baby blues are more common in primiparas.

- **Postpartum depression** is clinical depression that lasts 1 to 6 weeks.

  - Physiological changes with birth trigger a major depression.
  - Women with a history of depression are at higher risk.
  - Untreated, it can compromise the baby's socialization and emotional health.
  - This requires referral to a caregiver for evaluation and treatment.
  - The Edinburgh Postnatal Depression Scale helps in detection (see Figure 1-1). A score of 10 or more may indicate possible depression of varying severity.

ADVICE TO CLINICIANS
BE ALERT!

Red flags for potential postpartum depression in a mother:

▶ She lacks confidence in her ability to breastfeed, with a possible drop in milk production.
▶ She says she is lonely and has no visitors and no place to go.
▶ She does not answer the telephone or stays away from home in an attempt to keep busy.
▶ She lacks tolerance for other family members.
▶ She seems detached from her baby and does not refer to her baby by name.
▶ She worries that something is not "right."
▶ She entertains thoughts of harming herself—this requires urgent evaluation by a psychiatrist.

Edinburgh Postnatal Depression Scale (EPDS)

Instructions for users:

The mother is asked to underline the response that comes closest to how she has been feeling in the previous 7 days. All 10 items must be completed. Care should be taken to avoid the possibility of the mother discussing her answers with others. The mother should complete the scale herself, unless she has limited English or has difficulty with reading. The EPDS may be used at 6–8 weeks to screen postnatal women. The child health clinic, postnatal checkup, or a home visit may provide suitable opportunities for its completion.

Name: _____   Baby's Age: _____

Address: _____

As you have recently had a baby, we would like to know how you are feeling. Please UNDERLINE the answer that comes closest to how you have felt IN THE PAST 7 DAYS, not just how you feel today.

1. I have been able to laugh and see the funny side of things.
   a. As much as I always could – 0
   b. Not quite so much now –1
   c. Definitely not so much now – 2
   d. Not at all – 3
2. I have looked forward with enjoyment to things.
   a. As much as I ever did – 0
   b. Rather less than I used to – 1
   c. Definitely less than I used to – 2
   d. Hardly at all – 3
*3. I have blamed myself unnecessarily when things went wrong.
   a. Yes, most of the time – 3
   b. Yes, some of the time – 2
   c. Not very often – 1
   d. No, never – 0
4. I have been anxious or worried for no good reason.
   a. No, not at all – 0
   b. Hardly ever – 1
   c. Yes, sometimes – 2
   d. Yes, very often – 3
*5. I have felt scared or panicky for not very good reason.
   a. Yes, quite a lot – 3
   b. Yes, sometimes – 2
   c. No, not much – 1
   d. No, not at all – 0

*6. Things have been getting on top of me.
    a. Yes, most of the time I haven't been able to cope at all – 3
    b. Yes, sometimes I haven't been coping as well as usual – 2
    c. No, most of the time I have coped quite well – 1
    d. No, I have been coping as well as ever – 0
*7. I have been so unhappy that I have had difficulty sleeping.
    a. Yes, most of the time – 3
    b. Yes, quite often – 2
    c. Not very often – 1
    d. No, not at all – 0
*8. I have felt sad or miserable.
    a. Yes, most of the time – 3
    b. Yes, quite often – 2
    c. Not very often – 1
    d. No, not at all – 0
*9. I have been so unhappy that I have been crying.
    a. Yes, most of the time – 3
    b. Yes, quite often – 2
    c. Only occasionally – 1
    d. No, never – 0
*10. The thought of harming myself has occurred to me.
    a. Yes, quite often – 3
    b. Sometimes – 2
    c. Hardly ever – 1
    d. Never – 0

Response categories are scored 0, 1, 2, and 3 according to increased severity of the symptoms. Items marked with an asterisk are reverse scored (i.e., 3, 2, 1, and 0). The total score is calculated by adding together the scores for each of the 10 items. Users may reproduce the scale without further permission providing they respect copyright by quoting the names of the authors, the title, and the source of the paper in all reproduced copies.

Figure 1-1 Edinburgh Postnatal Depression Scale.
Source: Coz, L. L., Holden, J. M., and Sagovsky, R. (1987). "Detection of Postnatal Depression: Development of the 10-Item Edinburgh Postnatal Depression Scale." *British Journal of Psychiatry* 150:782–786.

- **Postpartum psychosis** occurs in 1 to 2 out of 1000 women.
  - The mother feels a loss of control, rational thought, and social functioning.
  - The mother has overwhelming delusions and hallucinations.
  - The mother may attempt suicide or harm the child—this requires urgent evaluation by a psychiatrist.

ADVICE TO CLINICIANS
BE ALERT!

Symptoms of postpartum depression:

▶ Mood changes

▶ Loss of pleasure

▶ Poor concentration

▶ Low self-esteem

▶ Guilt at failing as a mother and wife

▶ Sleep disturbances

▶ Fatigue

▶ Flat affect in voice tone

▶ Loss of appetite

Survivors of Sexual Abuse

- Incidence of sexual abuse ranges from 7% to 36% of women and 3% to 29% of men.

    - It affects the functioning of at least 20% of adult survivors.
    - It predisposes women to major depression or post-traumatic stress disorder.

- Pregnancy and childbirth are common times for remembering abuse.

    - The mother experiences the sounds or feelings of giving birth.
    - The mother is uncomfortable having the baby at her breast.
    - The mother feels a loss of control in the early days of parenting.
    - The mother is uncomfortable at the sight of milk during letdown.

- Memories, flashbacks, and emotions may interfere with the ability to breastfeed.

    - Early postpartum is the most stressful time, when a mother feels tired and vulnerable.
    - If nighttime breastfeeding is difficult, someone can feed her milk to the baby for those feeds.
    - Breastfeeding may be difficult when the baby gets older and more playful.
    - The mother may find breastfeeding to be healing or she may be unable to continue.

- Signs of possible past abuse:

    - Late prenatal care
    - Substance abuse
    - Mental health concerns
    - Eating disorders

ADVICE TO CLINICIANS
SEEK HELP

▶ Refer a mother for professional help if baby blues last beyond 2 weeks.

▶ Refer a sexual abuse survivor for professional help.

- Poor compliance with self-care
- Sexual dysfunction
- Feeding expressed milk with a bottle and not putting the baby to breast

Adjusting as a Couple

- Emotional adjustments:

    - The need for sexual adjustment is normal and common to new parents.
    - Some women have little desire for intimacy in the early weeks or months after giving birth.
    - The mother's breasts may be overly sensitive or unresponsive to foreplay.
    - Either partner may be reluctant to engage in foreplay that involves the breasts.
    - Increased sensuality is common and normal when breastfeeding the baby.

- Physical adjustments:

    - Physicians usually recommend abstaining from intercourse for 6 weeks postpartum.
    - Hormones decrease vaginal lubrication; the use of a water-soluble lubricant will help.
    - Recovery from birth interventions can interfere with the desire for intimacy.
    - Stretched pelvic floor muscles may decrease physical sensations; Kegel exercises will help.
    - Oxytocin released during orgasm can cause milk to let down; feed the baby before intercourse and absorb milk with a towel.
    - Adjust positioning to alleviate discomfort from an incision or full breasts.

Menstruation and Fertility

- Hormones during lactation disrupt the ovulation and menstrual cycle.

    - Some women produce a scanty show before their menstrual cycles resume.
    - Menstruation causes no significant changes in the composition of the mother's milk.
    - Altered taste of the milk may cause the baby to be fussy or refuse to breastfeed.

- Contraception:

    - The lactational amenorrhea method offers 98% protection with three conditions:

        ‣ Menses has not returned.
        ‣ The baby is breastfed exclusively without significant amounts of other foods and with no bottles or pacifiers that would replace suckling at the breast.
        ‣ The baby is younger than 6 months of age.

- Natural family planning:

  - The woman charts basal body temperature or checks vaginal secretions.
  - Changes in cervical mucus before ovulation help signal the beginning of fertile days.
  - The couple abstains from sex during fertile days.
  - Patterns early in lactation may be less clearly defined than after regular cycles resume.

- Oral contraceptives:

  - Breastfeeding women should delay hormonal contraceptives until 6 weeks postpartum.
  - Those with estrogen and progesterone may lower production and composition of milk.
  - Progestin-only oral contraceptives may interfere with milk production.

- Intrauterine devices (IUDs):

  - Nonhormonal IUDs do not seem to affect lactation.
  - Progesterone-releasing IUDs may decrease milk production.

- Other contraceptive methods:

  - A vaginal ring contains estrogen; a nonestrogen alternative may be a better choice.
  - The implant Levonorgestrel releases progesterone.
  - Depo-Provera may impair milk supply; delay its use until lactation is established.
  - The Patch contains estrogen and progesterone.
  - Barrier methods such as a condom, diaphragm, cervical cap, and spermicidal do not interfere with lactation.
  - Tubal ligation immediately postpartum can increase pain, and IV fluids can cause edema.

Parenting

- Encourage parents to be active and informed health consumers.

  - Informed consent requires sufficient information and education.
  - Parents have a *right* to the information necessary in making an informed choice.
  - Caregivers have a *responsibility* to inform parents of healthy choices.

- Couples acquire the parental role in stages:

  - Anticipatory stage: Take classes, read books, subscribe to parenting and childcare magazines, and ask family and friends about parenting.

ADVICE TO CLINICIANS
BE ALERT!

Caution parents about dangerous parenting programs or practices.

▷ Baby-training programs can cause low milk supply, low infant weight gain, baby rejecting the breast, and premature weaning.
▷ Present information from reliable medical sources.
▷ Document concerns regarding a baby's health or a mother's milk production.
▷ Urge parents to have frequent weight checks for their baby.

- Formal stage: Begin to view parenting more personally and strive for perfection.
- Informal stage: Modify and blend individual roles to fit their family.
- Personal stage: Parenting style evolves to be consistent with their personalities and in response to the needs of their baby, their family backgrounds, and the couple's interaction.

Opposition from Others

- Opposition from the baby's father influences a mother's decision to breastfeed. Possible responses:

  - He believes the baby will be too dependent on the mother: meeting a child's present needs will make him less dependent in the future.
  - He believes breastfeeding will interfere with their sex life: having a baby interferes with all parents' sex lives no matter how they feed their baby.
  - He feels jealous or left out of the baby's care: plan special time alone as a couple and suggest ways to be involved other than with feedings.

ADVICE TO CLINICIANS
BE EMPOWERING

▷ Form a partnership with parents.
▷ Help parents become informed health consumers.
▷ Place control and power with the mother and baby, not the caregiver.
▷ Encourage parents to be independent, self-reliant, and accountable for their choices.
▷ Help mothers verbalize feelings, take in information, and join in problem solving.
▷ Boost a mother's confidence, validate concerns, and point out positive things about her baby.
▷ Encourage parents to network formally and informally with other parents.

- He is concerned about the well-being of his partner and baby: breastfeeding contributes to family harmony and enhances a baby's disposition, growth, and development.
- He regards the mother's breasts as only sexual: discuss this with sensitivity and understanding.
- He questions breastfeeding when their baby gets older: breastfeeding has nutritional and developmental benefits at any age.

- Grandmothers often have a pivotal role in a mother's breastfeeding.

  - Explain that she is doing what is best for her child, just as her mother did with the information available to her at the time.

    ▶ She may see the daughter's choice to breastfeed as a reflection on her own parenting.
    ▶ She may believe breastfeeding makes the strains of early parenting more difficult.
    ▶ She may not want her daughter to have the same disappointment and failure she did.
    ▶ She may be envious that her daughter can do something she was not able to do.

  - Explain breastfeeding patterns and dispel misconceptions.

    ▶ Babies should be breastfed for at least 1 year or longer.
    ▶ Putting a baby to bed with a bottle is unsafe and causes tooth decay.
    ▶ Feeding cereal in the bottle can cause the baby to choke.
    ▶ Babies should not receive solid foods before they are 4–6 months old.
    ▶ Placing the baby on his back to sleep helps prevent SIDS.
    ▶ Babies should not be exposed to secondhand smoke.

- Minimize the potential for comments from strangers by breastfeeding discreetly in public.
- Educate friends and develop friendships with supportive people.
- Consider whether an unsupportive physician will work for her.

> **ADVICE TO CLINICIANS**
> **BE EMPOWERING**
>
> Support women who experience opposition to breastfeeding.
>
> ▶ Provide extra contact, confidence building, and anticipatory guidance.
> ▶ Provide research articles if opposition is from a physician.
> ▶ Suggest reading material if opposition is from the baby's father, another relative, or a friend.
> ▶ Refer mothers to a breastfeeding support group.
> ▶ Help mothers cope without making judgments or becoming overly involved.

Helping Siblings Adjust to a New Baby

- Prepare the older child for the baby's arrival.

  - Explain how a fetus develops and what the mother will do at doctor visits and in the hospital.
  - Look at family baby pictures and read books that show a new baby in the family.
  - Have the child help with baby items and with packing the mother's suitcase.
  - Change sleeping arrangements early and in a way the child does not feel crowded out.
  - Collect pictures to show a mother in the hospital, coming home, and at home with the baby.
  - Explain what babies do and how family activities will change; visit a family with a baby.
  - Visit the hospital with the older child during the pregnancy; take a sibling class and a tour.
  - If the sibling is present at the baby's birth, have a caregiver available to meet the child's needs.

- Help the child adjust to the new baby.

  - Help the child feel special in new ways.

    - Give the mother's undivided attention the first time she sees him following the birth.
    - Create situations where each child can look at, touch, or hold the baby.
    - Set aside special moments each day for the other child individually.

  - Incorporate the older child into feedings.

    - Use the football hold to facilitate having the child next to the mother.
    - Engage the child during feedings with books, games, and other activities.
    - Be sensitive to the child's possible renewed interest in breastfeeding.

  - Be sensitive to the older child's need for attention.

    - The child may whine or use baby talk.
    - The child may wake during the night, cling to the mother, or hit the baby.
    - A previously toilet-trained child may wet the bed.

Lifestyle Factors

Single Mother

- She has sole responsibility for the baby.
- She may live alone and juggle job, schooling, household responsibilities, and parenting.

- She may live with parents, trying to maintain an identity as a family unit with her baby.
- Emotional stress and demands can cause missed feedings and lowered milk production.
- She may lack the desire or time to prepare nutritious meals.

Teen Mother

- She may lack sound prenatal care and nutrition.
- She may feel inadequate as a parent.
- She may be engaged in a power struggle with her mother.
- She may not breastfeed often enough to produce a robust supply.
- She may find it difficult to overcome problems to continue breastfeeding.
- She needs a one-to-one relationship with someone who cares about her.
- She needs others to treat her as an adult.
- She needs consistency and simple, clear information.

Same Sex Couples

- The baby may be adopted and the mother wants to establish a milk supply.
- Be honest with regard to options.
- Support the parents with a nonjudgmental attitude.

Older Primigravida

- These mothers are often set in their ways and have higher education and high expectations.
- They may have difficulty adapting to motherhood.
- They are typically more fatigued and stressed.
- They may find it difficult to make decisions and need more support.

Cultural Differences

- Learning about cultural characteristics enhances sensitivity to clients' cultural beliefs.

ADVICE TO CLINICIANS
BE EMPOWERING

Learn community demographics to assist in interactions with families.

▶ Recognize unchangeable factors such as personality or lifestyle limitations.
▶ Respond appropriately to customs and body language.
▶ Ask about etiquette in a situation if you are unsure of cultural customs.
▶ Accept health and illness behaviors that do not compromise breastfeeding.

- Degree of acculturation determines how firmly women cling to traditional values.
- Existence of contradictory values can create confusion.
- Cultural heritage and economic standing will influence how long a woman breastfeeds.

- Learn about cultural customs for breastfeeding and infant care.

  - New mothers do not consume cold foods and beverages for several weeks or months.
  - Limitations are placed on postpartum activity for new mothers.
  - There are taboos on ways of touching or referring to the baby.
  - Colostrum is considered valueless or undesirable and breastfeeding is discouraged until the second or third postpartum day.
  - The role of the baby's father may differ culturally.

Low-Income Mothers

- Low income affects healthcare choices.

  - Lower educational and occupational levels and self-esteem can lead to limited expectations.
  - Women often live in unfavorable housing conditions with inadequate community services.
  - Physical and mental health problems may be prevalent.
  - Broken families and relocation problems can create obstacles.
  - Women often experience isolation, alienation, or language differences.
  - Childbirth class participation may be low because of cost, availability, or lack of interest.
  - Women may have multiple sites for prenatal care, birth, and family health care.

- Low-income women often face psychosocial challenges.

  - They may lack accurate information and family and community support.
  - Breastfeeding may seem like one more potential stress or failure in their lives.
  - They may face crises and challenges related to survival.
  - There may be little discretionary time or money.
  - There may be concerns about pain, smoking, and returning to work.
  - They may feel detached and unable to control their lives and surroundings.
  - They may distrust the "system" that healthcare providers represent.
  - They may be unaware of community resources available to low-income women.

- Factors that increase the likelihood of breastfeeding:

  - Women who have a higher level of education, are married, and have greater ego maturity

- Family and peer support, particularly when someone close to her had a positive breastfeeding experience
- Community health interventions
- Encouragement from medical personnel
- Peer support through discussion groups

Working Mothers
The Decision to Combine Working and Breastfeeding

- Women likely to combine work and breastfeeding share common traits.

  - They are older and more educated.
  - They work fewer hours per week and occupy positions at a more professional level.
  - They return to work later than 2 to 3 months postpartum.

- Women may be unaware it is possible to continue breastfeeding.

  - A nonsupportive society presents obstacles.
  - Health professionals send mixed messages.
  - They have a short maternity leave.
  - They lack breastfeeding knowledge.
  - They view breastfeeding as an interruption in career and lifestyle.
  - Society views employment as a socially acceptable reason to wean.

- An unsupportive work environment may not accommodate breastfeeding.

  - It does not allow space and protected time for milk expression.
  - The employer does not support breastfeeding.
  - Colleagues are resentful.
  - The mother faces potential demotion, job loss, verbal abuse, or social isolation. *Maternity Protection Kit: A Breastfeeding Perspective* is available from the International Lactation Consultant Association (ILCA).

ADVICE TO CLINICIANS
SEEK HELP

- ▶ Refer low-income women to community resources such as Women, Infants, and Children (WIC) in the United States and Canada Prenatal Nutrition Program (CPNP).
- ▶ Enlist help from other women in the culture to promote breastfeeding.
- ▶ Access bilingual help through a colleague, friend or relative of the mother, or a local school.
- ▶ Enlist a female interpreter who communicates accurately with no personal opinions or values.

Making It Work

- Encourage women to explore options and support at work.

  - Determine employer, supervisor, and coworkers' breastfeeding knowledge and support.
  - Extend maternity leave and insurance coverage for lactation assistance or a breast pump.
  - Return part-time for days per week or hours per day; alter, reduce, or eliminate hours.
  - Arrange job sharing, telecommuting from home, or flexible hours.
  - Arrange childcare that will keep the mother and child together or near one another.
  - Return at the end of the workweek to minimize feeling overwhelmed in the transition.

- Arrange childcare that accommodates breastfeeding.

  - Decide whether the baby will receive the mother's milk exclusively.

    - Nurse on breaks throughout the day if childcare is available onsite or nearby.
    - Increase feedings when the mother and baby are together (**reverse cycle nursing**).
    - Express milk for missed feedings to feed to the baby during the mother's absence.
    - Feed artificial baby milk during the separation and nurse when with the baby.

  - Begin preparations 2 to 3 weeks before returning to work.

    - Practice milk expression and begin storing milk.
    - Practice the feeding method when the baby is not too hungry.
    - Have a familiar person feed the baby.
    - Warm the bottle nipple to make it more acceptable to the baby.
    - Ease into a feeding routine that mimics the work schedule.
    - Make trial runs with the childcare provider.

  - Acquaint the childcare provider with needs related to breastfeeding.

    - Provide written instructions about the care of the mother's milk.
    - Explain preferences such as wanting the baby to be hungry when the mother returns.
    - Review the baby's feeding regimen and method.
    - Watch for signs of hunger so the baby does not become overly hungry.
    - Hold the baby in the same position as for breastfeeding.
    - Pace feedings and put the baby in charge of drawing milk into his mouth.

  ▸ Communicate closely about feedings.

    – Amount the baby takes at a feeding.
    – How the baby handles the feeding method.
    – How the baby is doing in general.

- Prepare for breastfeeding issues after returning to work.

  ▪ Express milk regularly to maintain milk production.

    ▸ Respond to breast fullness.
    ▸ Avoid engorgement, mastitis, plugged ducts, or excessive leaking.
    ▸ Match pumping breaks to the baby's feeding schedule.
    ▸ Pump 10 to 15 minutes at each pumping session with a double electric breast pump.

  ▪ Take measures to relax when pumping.

    ▸ Perform breast massage and apply moist heat.
    ▸ Play a tape of the baby's sounds.
    ▸ Keep a picture and article of the baby's clothing nearby.

  ▪ Preserve the safety of the milk.

    ▸ Store the milk in quantities the baby will take at one feeding.
    ▸ Milk can remain at room temperature for up to 6 hours.
    ▸ Cool and transfer the milk to the refrigerator at home.

  ▪ Wear appropriate clothing.

    ▸ Wear clothes with easy breast access for pumping and for nursing before and after work.
    ▸ Wear breast pads to absorb leaking; keep a jacket, sweater, or change of clothes at work.

  ▪ Plan quiet time with the baby at the end of the workday.
  ▪ The baby may increase the frequency and duration of feedings when with the mother.

Employer Support for Breastfeeding

- Benefits to employers:

  ▪ There is a cost savings of $3 for every $1 invested in breastfeeding support.
  ▪ Breastfed children of employees experience less illness.
  ▪ Breastfeeding mothers have less absenteeism to care for ill children.
  ▪ Healthcare costs are lower (average of $400 less per baby over the first year).

Features of an employer lactation room:

▶ An accessible location with privacy, a lockable door, and a privacy screen
▶ Access to a nearby clean and safe water source
▶ A sink for washing hands and rinsing breast pump equipment
▶ Access to hygienic storage alternatives for storing expressed milk
▶ Comfortable chairs with arm support
▶ A table or desk for the breast pump, the baby's picture, a beverage, clock, telephone, and other items
▶ A sign-in book to track feedback and the number of employees who use the space
▶ Options for passing time such as quiet music and reading material
▶ A refrigerator for storing the mother's milk
▶ A mirror for checking that clothes are back in place before leaving the room

- Employee productivity improves, and morale and loyalty are greater.
- Employers can attract and retain valuable employees.
- Employers have a family-friendly image in the community.

• Breastfeeding-friendly employer practices:

- Extend the length of paid maternity leave.
- Provide childcare at or near the work site.
- Provide prenatal and postpartum programs for parents.
- Protect pumping time and prohibit nonsupport or sexual harassment from other employees.
- Allow mothers to take breastfeeding breaks and bring their babies to work.

Tutorial for Students and Interns

Key Clinical Management Strategies

From *Clinical Guidelines for the Establishment of Exclusive Breastfeeding*, ILCA, 2005:

• Include family members or significant others in breastfeeding education.
• Provide anticipatory guidance for common problems that can interfere with exclusive breastfeeding.
• Discuss contraceptive options and their possible effect on milk production.

Key Clinical Competencies

From *Clinical Competencies for IBCLC Practice* available at www.iblce.org:

☐ Provide individualized breastfeeding care with an emphasis on the mother's ability to make informed decisions.

☐ Assess mother's psychological state and provide information appropriate to her situation.

☐ Include those family members or friends the mother identifies as significant to her.

☐ Report instances of child abuse or neglect to specific agencies as mandated or appropriate.

☐ Instruct the mother about family planning methods and their relationship to breastfeeding.

☐ Demonstrate knowledge of and sensitivity to cultural differences.

☐ Assist mothers with cultural beliefs that are not evidence based and may interfere with breastfeeding.

☐ Assist adolescent mothers.

☐ Assist mothers with strategies for returning to school or work.

☐ Assist mothers with postpartum psychological issues including transient sadness ("baby blues") and postpartum depression.

☐ Make appropriate referrals to other healthcare professionals and community resources.

☐ Obtain clinical experience with breastfeeding hotlines and warm lines.

☐ Obtain clinical experience with a volunteer community support group meeting.

From Theory to Practice

1. How would you describe health consumerism to a mother?
2. How does informed consent relate to health consumerism?
3. What distinguishes medical advice from parenting advice? What are some examples of parenting advice in counseling breastfeeding mothers?
4. Why does a mother need to be honest with her healthcare providers if she chooses not to follow their advice?
5. What factors might affect a low-income mother's motivation to breastfeed?
6. What special needs might a single mother have with breastfeeding?
7. How can you empower a teen mother to breastfeed for an extended time?
8. How can you learn a woman's cultural influence on breastfeeding and mothering practices?
9. What cultural practices could be detrimental to breastfeeding and how would you approach this with a mother?
10. What options are there in accommodating breastfeeding for a woman who plans to return to work?
11. What preparations related to breastfeeding will help to facilitate a smooth transition for returning to work?

12. What benefits are there to the employer who supports breastfeeding?
13. How would you distinguish between postpartum blues, depression, and psychosis?

Consider what you would investigate and how you would respond to these statements by a mother. What would be your first statement to her?

14. I feel so out of control with my emotions since my baby was born last week. I never know whether to laugh or cry!
15. My older children are constantly getting on my nerves. The baby is 2 months old, and breastfeeding still takes up so much of my time. I don't know how much more I can take.
16. My baby is 1 month old, and I am constantly tired. Breastfeeding seems to be taking a lot out of me.
17. My husband doesn't seem very interested in our baby. He seems to resent all the time I spend breastfeeding.
18. My sister breastfed for 18 months and didn't get pregnant even though she wasn't using any form of birth control. I plan to do the same thing.
19. My mother-in-law is always telling me I don't have enough milk and that my baby seems hungry all the time. My husband says to just ignore her.
20. My 2-year-old daughter is jealous of the time I spend nursing my new baby and is disruptive during feedings.
21. I don't have time to express milk at work. I'm away from my baby for 9 hours, I leak all the time, and my breasts are uncomfortable. And I don't have enough milk in the freezer for my caregiver to keep giving my milk to my baby.

CHAPTER 2

Communication and Teaching

In This Chapter

Communication

The Spoken Word

- Words contribute 7% to the message conveyed.
- The word *but* negates the first half of a thought; connect two thoughts with *and* instead.
- The word *should* implies the other person was doing something inappropriately or incorrectly.
- Avoid words that create negative images, such as *inadequate* or *unsuccessful*.
- Avoid phrases that confuse mothers or send mixed messages.

Voice Tone

- Voice tone contributes 38% to the message conveyed.
- Achieve a comfortable volume and rate of speech.
- Control the pitch of your voice.

Body Language

- Body language contributes 55% to the message conveyed.
- A pleasant facial expression creates a warm and inviting atmosphere.
- Eye contact conveys a desire to communicate.
- Open body posture and leaning forward shows your intent to communicate on a meaningful level.

- A comfortable distance between two people is with one not too far away and not too close to another.
- Placing the mother at an equal or greater height promotes her importance.
- The touch of a hand, or an arm placed around someone's shoulder, can convey warmth, caring, and encouragement. Ask permission before touching a mother or baby.

Counseling Skills
Listening

- Listening involves perceiving with your ears, eyes, and imagination.
- Validate feelings, emotions, and concerns through attending, active listening, empathetic listening, reassuring, praising, and building hope.
- Avoid active participation early in the contact in order to gather sufficient information and insights.
- Levels of listening are ignoring (the lowest level), pretending, selective listening, and attentive listening (the highest level).
- Passive listening (attending) moves the conversation along with vocalization or body language.
- Active listening gathers information, clarifies messages, shows acceptance, and encourages a response.
- Empathetic listening helps the listener to understand emotionally and to work through feelings.

Facilitating

- Offering reassurance, building hope, and identifying strengths influence the mother positively.
- Asking open-ended questions, rather than closed questions, elicits more information: *Who, what, when, where, why, how, how much,* and *how often.*
- Clarifying, interpreting, focusing, and summarizing elicit more information, help to define the situation, and focus on specific concerns.
- Take time to gain the mother's trust and clarify the situation before beginning problem solving.
- Gather enough information so problem solving is not premature or incorrect.

Problem Solving

- Problem solving helps in gaining control and is pivotal to producing the desired response.
- Help mothers with immediate physical comfort before problem solving.
- Give parents information at the appropriate time to help them grow as parents.

- Correct misconceptions or mismanagement with sensitivity.
- Use a nonassertive approach to encourage the mother to participate in problem solving.
- Recognize when a problem requires in-person rather than telephone help.
- Check for hidden factors that may contribute to the problem before forming a hunch.
- Form a hunch based on information and impressions you gained.
- Be open to new information that may lead you to form a new hunch.
- Explore alternative hunches until you and the mother define the problem.
- Develop a plan with the mother as an equal partner and ask her to repeat the plan.

Follow-Up

- Arrange appropriate follow-up after every contact.
- Plan and arrange for the next contact.
- Make sure the mother knows when she may call you.
- Evaluate how the session went and what else you could have done.
- Seek outside resources as needed.

Education
Adult Learning

- Create an effective learning climate.

  - Motivation to satisfy a need or goal is a stimulus to learning.
  - Active involvement in learning will depend on the level of motivation.
  - Reinforcement increases the likelihood that a specific response will occur in the future.
  - Repetition increases the strength of an association and slows the process of forgetting.
  - Processing of information depends on cognitive ability and complexity of the information.
  - Ability to form mental images influences the degree of recall.
  - Reinforce verbal instruction with written materials, demonstrations, and other visual aids.
  - Avoid overwhelming mothers with too much information.
  - Use humor as a learning tool.

    - The use of humor enhances learning.
    - Humor evolves naturally in a relaxed climate of support and acceptance.
    - Humor stimulates alertness and memory, and enhances learning and creativity.

COMMUNICATION AND TEACHING

- Individualize your approach with each mother.

  - What is her learning style?
  - What does she need to learn?
  - Is she ready to learn?
  - What will she respond to?

- Serve as a facilitator and actively involve the mother.

  - *Tell me and I may remember*: The lowest involvement, appropriate for verbal instruction that does not require visual or interactive reinforcement.
  - *Show me and I may understand*: Higher involvement, with demonstration enhancing learning.
  - *Involve me and I may master*: The highest involvement, with return demonstration enhancing learning.

- Make positive impressions on learners.

  - Display self-confidence.
  - Show a desire and ability to share knowledge and relate to people.
  - Be flexible and adapt.
  - Be enthusiastic with a sense of humor and comfortable tone of informality.
  - Display a strong knowledge base and respect for the learner.
  - Maintain frequent eye contact, positive body language, and neat, clean, and stylish attire.
  - Speak with a strong voice and carefully pronounced words.

Health benefits of laughter:

- ▶ It speeds up heart rate and raises blood pressure.
- ▶ It accelerates breathing and increases oxygen consumption.
- ▶ It stimulates muscles and relaxes muscle tension.
- ▶ It reduces pain and anxiety.
- ▶ It stimulates the cardiovascular system.
- ▶ It stimulates the sympathetic nervous system.
- ▶ It stimulates production of catecholamines and endorphins.
- ▶ It increases adrenaline in the brain.

Educating Mothers

- Recognize learning needs and capitalize on teachable moments.
- Keep it simple.

  - Communicate clearly.
  - Offer the simplest, least complicated explanation in lay terms.
  - Relate information in a friendly and low-key manner.
  - Avoid overwhelming a mother or making her appear uninformed.

- Relate only information that is up to date, correct, and evidence based.

- Check for accuracy if there is conflicting information.
- Teach practical information.
- Point out options.
- Offer useful suggestions.
- Explain why and how a technique works.
- Explain reasons behind your suggestions.

• Reinforce learning with handouts, demonstrations, and other visual aids.

Prenatal Teaching

• Help parents make an informed infant feeding decision.

  ▪ Over half of women make their infant feeding choice before pregnancy.

    ◗ The most likely breastfeeders are in their midthirties, college educated, white, married, and are middle income.
    ◗ Women least likely to breastfeed are blacks and teens, though rates are increasing.
    ◗ Breastfeeders perceive breastfeeding as more convenient.
    ◗ Bottle feeders perceive breastfeeding as less convenient.

  ▪ Several factors influence a woman's decision.

    ◗ The baby's father is pivotal to the decision; encourage fathers to participate in classes. Attitude and knowledge level of caregivers greatly influence decisions and confidence.

ADVICE TO CLINICIANS
TEACH EFFECTIVELY

Focus on a few key points at the heart of the message without overwhelming mothers.

  ▶ Speak slowly and clearly, and give simple explanations.
  ▶ Enlist resources to communicate with mothers who have language differences (see the Spanish/French glossary in Appendix I).
  ▶ Provide resources for mothers who are deaf, blind, or of diminished mental ability.
  ▶ Offer specific, practical suggestions rather than general ones.
  ▶ Reinforce verbal explanations with visual aids and return demonstrations.
  ▶ Provide a checklist of what you and the mother discuss.
  ▶ Ask the mother to repeat instructions to ensure that she understands them.
  ▶ Try to get feedback to indicate the mother will act on the suggestions.
  ▶ Offer attractive, simply written and illustrated brochures at an appropriate reading level.

  ▶ Commercial messages about artificial baby milk imply little difference with human milk.
  ▶ The media promotes sexual images of breasts.

- Help women address personal barriers to breastfeeding.

  - They may feel embarrassed nursing in front of others.
  - Work or school routines may create conflicts.
  - Lack of confidence or fear of being totally responsible for their baby's weight gain and health may create worries.
  - Lifestyle issues such as diet, stress, substance abuse, and inadequate sleep may interfere.
  - A need for control or customs in the home environment may present challenges.
  - They may be uncomfortable having a baby at the breast (common in survivors of sexual or physical abuse).
  - They may lack support from family or friends.

- Teach women how to prepare for breastfeeding (see prenatal breastfeeding class in Figure 2-1).

  - Women with a history of preterm labor, miscarriage, or false labor should avoid nipple stimulation.
  - Encourage attendance at a breastfeeding class.

- Answer questions about selecting the baby's physician.

  - Confidence in and a working relationship with their physician are important to parents.
  - Mothers can ask about the physician's background, hospital affiliation, accessibility, breastfeeding knowledge, and standing orders.
  - Encourage mothers to be open with their physician about their breastfeeding.
  - Avoid driving a wedge between a mother and her physician.
  - When recommending physicians, give at least 3 names with information about their breastfeeding practices and standing orders.

- Build rapport and establish trust so that mothers accept advice more readily.

  - The earlier a woman receives information, the longer she is likely to breastfeed.
  - Encourage initial learning before delivery so postpartum teaching is reinforcement.
  - Attentiveness and retention may be greater in the later months of pregnancy.
  - See Figure 2-2 for questions to ask pregnant women.

Outline for a Prenatal Breastfeeding Class

A. Welcome and introductions
B. Breast or bottle?
   1. What have you heard about breastfeeding?
   2. How were you fed?
   3. What does our culture say about artificial baby milk?
   4. What does our culture say about breasts?
C. Why should you breastfeed?
   1. Risks of *not* breastfeeding
   2. How breastfeeding protects your baby
   3. How breastfeeding protects the mother
D. Your breasts
   1. Changes in pregnancy
   2. During lactation
E. Your milk production
   1. Colostrum to mature milk
   2. Feeding frequency
   3. Draining the breast
F. Your baby
   1. Speaking your baby's language—feeding behavior and sleep states
   2. Your baby's nutritional needs and eating patterns
G. Overview of breastfeeding management: video
H. Getting started with breastfeeding
   1. Putting your baby to breast at birth
   2. Baby's and mother's comfort
   3. Positions for holding baby
   4. Positioning and latch
   5. Nonnutritive and nutritive sucking
   6. Stimulating a sleepy baby
I. Breastfeeding in the early weeks
   1. Breastfeeding pattern
   2. Mother's diet and rest
   3. Knowing your baby is getting enough milk
   4. Avoiding engorgement and plugged ducts
   5. Expressing and storing your milk
   6. Practices to avoid
   7. How to find help
J. Open discussion and questions

COMMUNICATION AND TEACHING

Figure 2-1 Outline for a Prenatal Breastfeeding Class

Questions About Breastfeeding to Ask Pregnant Women

Assessing a woman's need for breastfeeding education

- How does she feel about the prospect of breastfeeding?
- What practical knowledge does she have about breastfeeding?
- What prior experience or exposure does she have to breastfeeding?
- How many friends or relatives have breastfed?
- What reading has she done on breastfeeding? What videos has she seen?
- Has she attended a breastfeeding information class?
- Is she attending prepared childbirth classes?
- What has her physician discussed with her about breastfeeding?
- What has she done to prepare for breastfeeding?
- Has she checked for inverted nipples?
- What has she learned about breast care?
- What clothing does she have that will allow her baby easy access to her breast?
- What arrangements has she made for help at home?
- Has she arranged for rooming-in if she is delivering in a hospital?
- Is she interested in attending group discussions with other breastfeeding mothers?
- What are her specific questions or concerns?

Figure 2-2 Questions About Breastfeeding to Ask Pregnant Women

---

Postpartum Teaching and Support

- Consistent encouragement, help, and guidance increase breastfeeding rates.

  - Offer a postpartum breastfeeding class for new mothers (see Figure 2-3).
  - Encourage early follow-up after discharge to assess feeding effectiveness and answer questions.
  - Provide anticipatory guidance at times when retention is high and decision making occurs.
  - Arrange frequent contact during the early weeks postpartum, either personally or through referral to a support group.
  - Provide a hotline, warm line, or e-mail access to ensure contact with mothers.

- Share medical information appropriately.

  - Present information in a manner of educating, not prescribing, unless you have prescriptive authority.
  - Read from an up-to-date authoritative source.
  - Recommend that the mother consult her baby's physician.
  - Assure client privacy and confidentiality (follow HIPAA regulations in the United States).

Sample Outline for a Postpartum Breastfeeding Class

A. Welcome and introductions
B. Recommendations for continued breastfeeding
   1. Exclusive breastmilk
   2. Combining breastfeeding with complementary feedings
   3. Risks of routine supplementation
C. Milk production
   1. How to know your baby is getting enough milk
   2. Feeding frequency and duration
   3. Importance of milk removal for sustaining production
   4. Growth spurts
D. Milestones as your baby grows
   1. Social development
   2. Feeding patterns
   3. Sleep patterns
   4. Teething
   5. Toddler and tandem breastfeeding
   6. Weaning
E. Fitting breastfeeding into your lifestyle
   1. Resuming activities and including your baby
   2. Diet, rest, and exercise
   3. Breastfeeding in public
F. Returning to work or school
   1. Options and expectations
   2. Planning ahead
   3. How you will feed your baby
   4. Pumps and other devices
   5. Meeting challenges
G. Open discussion and problem solving
   1. Where to find breastfeeding help
   2. Individual problems

Figure 2-3 Sample Outline for a Postpartum Breastfeeding Class

---

Educating Staff

- Achieve a continuum of supportive breastfeeding care for mothers and babies.
- Teach others to help and to carry through with consistent care.
- Mentor and assist staff members clinically with mothers and babies.
- Present short breastfeeding updates at unit meetings.
- Energize staff and generate enthusiasm through seminars, workshops, or conferences.

Misconceptions about breastfeeding:

▶ *My baby will be too dependent if he breastfeeds*—Breastfed babies seem to display more independence because their parents respond to their needs.

▶ *Breastfeeding is too time consuming*—There is less work involved in breastfeeding than in bottle feeding.

▶ *My mother didn't have enough milk, so maybe I won't either*—Her mother's experience has no bearing on her ability to breastfeed.

▶ *My milk might not agree with my baby*—A mother's milk is ideally suited to her baby, and breastfed babies rarely experience negative reactions to their mother's milk.

▶ *My breasts are too small to breastfeed*—The size of a woman's breasts depends on fatty tissue, not functional breast tissue, and usually has little bearing on ability to produce sufficient milk.

▶ *I am too high-strung to breastfeed*—Breastfeeding can be calming because of the hormones activated by nursing and the added skin contact with the baby.

▶ *If I breastfeed, my diet will be too restricted*—Breastfeeding babies generally can tolerate the same foods the mother can tolerate. The only foods a mother may need to restrict are those that seem to produce signs of intolerance in her baby.

▶ *If I have a cesarean birth, I won't be able to breastfeed*—The type of birth a mother experiences has no effect on her ability to breastfeed.

▶ *Breastfeeding will drain my energies too much*—Caring for a newborn infant is tiring regardless of feeding method. Breastfeeding encourages a mother to relax during feeding times.

▶ *Breastfeeding mothers lose their figures and get sagging breasts*—Sagging results from pregnancy and loss of muscle tone as a woman ages, not because she breastfed. Caloric demands of breastfeeding can actually help mothers control their weight.

▶ *Artificial baby milk is just as healthy as human milk*—Human milk is a live substance. It provides immunities and antibacterial properties. Artificial baby milk does not.

▶ *Breastfeeding is essentially an alternative to infant formula*—Breastfeeding is a dynamic process, a bonding relationship between a mother and her baby, not simply infant food.

▶ *I'll have to wean before I return to work*—Mothers who are separated from their babies have many options. Many employers and insurance companies support employees who breastfeed, as it lowers absenteeism and insurance claims. WIC provides a breast pump for WIC participants who return to work or school.

Postpartum teaching points:

▶ Breastfeed exclusively and in response to feeding behavior.
▶ Learn signs of effective and poor attachment and how to position the baby effectively.
▶ Use more than one breastfeeding position.
▶ Support the breast for early feedings when necessary.
▶ Learn typical infant patterns.
▶ Learn how to stimulate a sleepy baby to nurse.
▶ Learn how to comfort a fussy baby for an effective feeding.
▶ Watch for signs that the baby wants to end a feeding.
▶ Watch for signs of adequate infant hydration and establishment of milk supply.
▶ Know whom to call with questions or concerns.

- Maintain a bulletin board with monthly updates and highlights of staff members.
- Post breastfeeding messages in the locker room or restroom.
- Conduct a needs assessment or quiz to whet appetites and get input from staff.

Tutorial for Students and Interns

Key Clinical Management Strategies

From *Clinical Guidelines for the Establishment of Exclusive Breastfeeding*, ILCA, 2005:

- Include family members or significant others in breastfeeding education.
- Provide anticipatory guidance for common problems that can interfere with exclusive breastfeeding.
- Provide appropriate breastfeeding education materials.

Key Clinical Competencies

From *Clinical Competencies for IBCLC Practice*, available at www.iblce.org:

☐ Demonstrate effective communication skills to maintain collaborative and supportive relationships.
☐ Identify factors that might affect communication (e.g., age, cultural or language differences, deafness, blindness, or mental ability).
☐ Demonstrate appropriate body language (e.g., position in relation to the other person, comfortable eye contact, or appropriate tone of voice for the setting).

COMMUNICATION AND TEACHING

☐ Elicit information using effective counseling techniques (e.g., asking open-ended questions, summarizing the discussion, and providing emotional support).

☐ Ascertain a mother's knowledge about and goals for breastfeeding.

☐ Use adult education principles to provide instruction that will meet the mother's needs.

☐ Select appropriate written information and other teaching aids.

☐ Assess a mother's psychological state and provide information appropriate to her situation.

☐ Develop an appropriate breastfeeding plan in concert with the mother and assist her to implement it.

☐ Evaluate effectiveness of the breastfeeding plan.

☐ Identify problems and assess contributing factors and etiology of problems.

☐ Assist mothers with appropriate referrals.

☐ Instruct the mother about community resources for assistance with breastfeeding.

☐ Instruct the mother about plans for follow-up care for breastfeeding questions and the infant's medical and mother's postpartum examinations.

☐ Obtain clinical experience with teaching prenatal and postpartum breastfeeding classes.

From Theory to Practice

1. Why is body language such an important factor in communicating with mothers?
2. How can you capitalize on body language to enhance your communication with mothers?
3. What is the most important goal in counseling a breastfeeding mother?
4. How can you use the different types of listening—attending, active listening, and empathetic listening—to maximize your effect with mothers?
5. How do open-ended questions help you gather information that will help you in your interactions with mothers?
6. How can you help to empower mothers during problem solving?
7. What are the possible consequences of failing to provide adequate follow-up?
8. What is the role of the facilitator in adult learning?
9. How can you individualize teaching to accommodate a particular mother?
10. Why is humor an important element in educating mothers?
11. How can you avoid overwhelming a mother when you are educating her?
12. What influences a woman's decision when deciding on an infant feeding method?
13. How can you help a woman address personal barriers she may have to breastfeeding?
14. What misconceptions have the greatest potential for turning a mother away from breastfeeding? How can you help to dispel the misconceptions?

15. What does a woman need to do prenatally to prepare for breastfeeding?
16. What are the benefits to having contact with women prenatally?
17. How does postpartum teaching differ from prenatal teaching with respect to breastfeeding?
18. How much do hospital staff need to know about breastfeeding, and how can you make sure they know it?

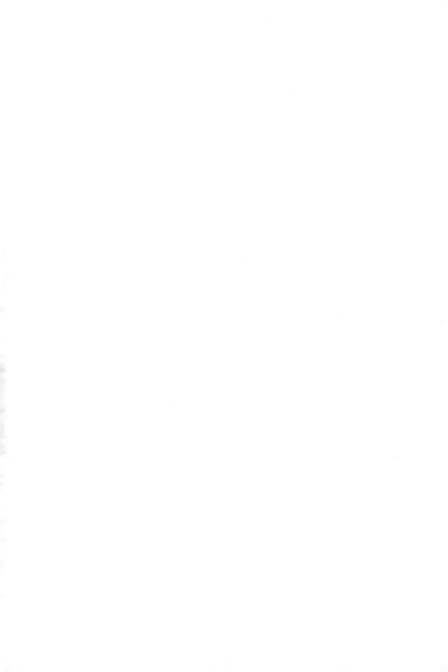

CHAPTER 3

Lactation Consultant Profession

In This Chapter

Practice Settings for Lactation Consultants

Hospital Practice

- Make rounds of mothers and assist with problems.
- Observe every mother breastfeed before discharge.
- Provide inpatient and staff education.
- Provide equipment and supplies for mothers.
- Provide discharge planning and refer mothers to support groups.
- See Appendix A for a sample job description.

Health Clinic or Women, Infants, and Children (WIC) Program

- Serve low-income mothers and infants.
- Counsel mothers with cultural, socioeconomic, and lifestyle differences.
- Teach classes and facilitate support groups.
- Teach and supervise peer counselors.

Physician Practice

- Assist pregnant women, mothers, and babies.
- Teach classes and facilitate support groups.

LACTATION CONSULTANT PROFESSION

35

- Make rounds of physician's patients in hospital.
- Provide follow-up calls and warm line.
- Patient load depends on physician's patient load.

Home Health Care

- Follow up with mothers after discharge.
- Assess the mother, baby, and breastfeeding.
- Provide anticipatory guidance on long-term issues.

Private Practice

- A seasoned IBCLC with extensive experience who sets up practice.
- Provide office and/or home visits and telephone follow-up.
- Document consultations, send physician reports, and retain records.
- Market the practice, and establish a referral base.
- Bill for services, and facilitate third-party reimbursement.

Professional Development

Formal Preparation

- Complete a lactation management program that covers the areas of the IBLCE blueprint.

  - Maternal and infant anatomy, physiology, and endocrinology
  - Maternal and infant nutrition, biochemistry, immunology, and infectious diseases
  - Maternal and infant pathology, pharmacology, and toxicology
  - Psychology, sociology, and anthropology

The IBCLC offers an adjunct service that builds on the physician–patient relationship.

- ▶ Communicate with primary care practitioners to establish yourself as part of the healthcare team.
- ▶ Share research and literature from disciplines that affect lactation and breastfeeding management.
- ▶ Share sound clinical information from unbiased sources.
- ▶ Help physicians recognize that mothers need support and validation in their decisions.
- ▶ Encourage physicians to refer mothers to an IBCLC.

- Growth parameters and developmental milestones
- Reading and interpretation of research
- Ethical and legal issues related to the practice of lactation consulting
- Technology related to breastfeeding
- Public health issues surrounding lactation

• Acquire clinical experience to apply theory and knowledge to clinical situations.

- Arrange for a mentor to guide you while you gain supervised experience.
- Enroll in a formal internship for supervised clinical experience.
- Acquire necessary clinical experience to qualify for IBCLC certification.

Role Acquisition

• Anticipatory stage

- You collect information from other lactation consultants, ILCA, IBLCE, providers of lactation education, and professional journals.
- You complete a comprehensive lactation management program.

• Formal stage

- You obtain clinical experience through an internship.
- Formal documents guide your practices.
- You begin to break down preconceived ideas and teachings.
- You choose from more than one method to determine your own practices.
- You practice rigidly and formally according to your perceived "rules" as you try to do everything right.
- You prefer the security of a mentor to guide you.

• Informal stage

- You begin to modify rigid rules and directions.
- You consider different approaches to care and weigh options.
- Interactions with mothers and other lactation consultants become more spontaneous.
- You have less fear of imperfection.

• Personal stage

- You develop a style that is consistent with your personality.
- You understand the motives and whims of new mothers and accept mothers' choices.
- You discard options if they are incompatible with your approach.
- You look critically at research and adapt it to your practice.
- You enjoy teaching others and assume leadership roles.

LACTATION CONSULTANT PROFESSION

Ethical Behavior

- Morals and ethics greatly influence social behavior.

  - Ethics are principles or standards of human conduct.
  - Moral customs change with each new generation, but ethical values are enduring.
  - Modern ethics teach that immediate pleasures must give way to a regard for ultimate good.

- In reality, no one practices ethical habits all the time.

  - We all have internal personal needs and external social needs.
  - We steer our lives by trial and error, and by intuition and reason.
  - Ethical values determine how we behave, how we treat one another, and how we enable others to thrive individually and collectively.

- Practice ethical behavior.

  - Treat others as unique individuals, value their worth, and treat them with respect.
  - Elicit the best from every person, and enable everyone to thrive.
  - Allow others to make choices and to be accountable for their mistakes.
  - Act with integrity, and keep commitments.
  - Be open, honest, caring, and responsive with others.
  - Educate yourself in order to grow both in wisdom and in your social life.
  - Remain true to your values and standards, without compromise.

Early theories on ethics:

▶ Pythagoras: The best life is one devoted to mental discipline.

▶ Sophists: Individual perception is valid only for oneself and cannot be generalized.

▶ Socrates: People will be virtuous if they know what virtue is.

▶ Greeks: The essence of virtue is self-control, which can be taught.

▶ Plato: Emotions should be subject to intellect and will.

▶ Aristotle: Moral virtues must accommodate differences among people and conditions.

▶ Stoics: Man should strive to be independent of material influences.

▶ Epicureans: Man should postpone immediate pleasure to attain lasting satisfaction in the future.

▶ Christianity: Man achieves goodness only with God's grace and not by will or intelligence.

▶ John Locke: Rational pursuit of happiness and pleasure leads to cooperation.

- Assure client privacy and confidentiality (follow HIPAA regulations in the United States)
- The IBLCE *Code of Ethics* guides lactation consultant practice (see Appendix C)

Maturing as a Lactation Consultant

Difficult Experiences

- A mother does not comply with your recommendations.

  - Give appropriate support and information.
  - Step back and respect the mother's choice.

- A mother or baby experiences medical complications.

  - Work through the grief process just as the mother does.

- A mother experiences external interference.

  - Educate the other person.
  - Be open and frank with the mother.
  - Provide follow-up care.

Professional Burnout

- Take measures to avoid burnout.

  - Accept your limitations.
  - Establish personal boundaries and make time for yourself and your family.
  - Network with colleagues, attend conferences, and become involved in professional activities.

- Signs of emotional burnout:

  - Tunnel vision
  - Loss of coping skills
  - Lack of focus and concentration
  - Unexplained physical pain
  - Fatigue
  - Irrational behavior, a feeling of being on an "emotional roller coaster"
  - Avoiding obligations and other avoidance behaviors
  - Feeling that life is out of control
  - Insomnia
  - Irritation
  - Depression
  - Inability to manage time

LACTATION CONSULTANT PROFESSION

Avoiding Pitfalls in Helping Mothers

- Accept your limitations.
- Avoid getting overly involved with mothers.
- Avoid discussing your own breastfeeding experience.
- Avoid making value judgments.
- Avoid interrupting others with your own comments.
- Avoid overwhelming mothers with too much information or technology.
- Avoid being too solution oriented.
- Provide follow-up.

Reading Research
Types of Research Articles

- **Editorials** are not studies and are not critically reviewed.
- **Case studies** report on a problem, diagnosis, or treatment and cannot be used to generalize.
- **Meta-analysis** combines data of several studies to test conclusions.
- **Reviews**, written by experts, analyze the best and worst studies with little or no original data.
- **Clinical practice** articles are reports of applications in real life.
- **Research** reports put long-held beliefs or new ideas to a scientific test.

Structure of Scientific Articles

- **Title:** Explains main findings and may be two sentences long.
- **Authors:** Tend to publish profusely in a specific, narrow discipline.
- **Abstract:** Is a brief summary that explain a study.
- **Introduction:** Contains the purpose, parameters, and restraints of the study.
- **Literature review:** Explains previous research.
- **Methods:** Describe how researchers operationalized the hypothesis, how subjects were recruited, tools used to measure outcomes, surveys, scales, tests, definition of terms, and statistical methods.
- **Results:** Often displayed in graphs, tables and charts, they are peer reviewed for accuracy.
- **Discussion:** Reviews reasons for the study and relevant literature, summarizes results, and suggests applications and further research.
- **References and bibliography:** List of the citations referred to in the article.

Study Design

- **Retrospective study:** Uses two comparison groups, with output variables describing the subjects after follow-up or treatment.

- **Prospective study:** Samples subjects based on input variables believed to influence outcomes.
- **Cross-sectional study:** Researchers gather data from everyone at the same time, relying on record keeping or memory.
- **Descriptive study:** Lists many relevant variables of a defined sample rather than comparing two groups.
- **Qualitative study:** Researchers observe subjects and events in a natural setting rather than establishing a control.
- **Randomized clinical trial:** Treatment groups are treated the same in all ways except for the treatment itself.
- **Blind clinical trial:** Knowledge of which treatment the patient received remains secret until analysis of the data begins.

Statistical Tests

- **Confidence intervals:** Determine statistical significance of a result, the range within which a population's true value is expected to be found.
- **Chi-square:** Determines whether proportions in two groups are significantly different; large chi-square values usually lead to low, statistically significant P values.
- **Cohen's kappa:** Shows that two observers who rate an event on a scale are in close agreement.
- **Cronbach's alpha test:** Determines reliability of an instrument.
- **Regression:** Determines the relationship between a predictor (independent) variable and an outcome (dependent) variable.
- **T test:** Decides between two contradictory hypotheses about the mean of a sample.
- **Odds ratio:** Summarizes relative proportion in two different groups.

Critical Reading of Research

- Look at the title and consider what you know about the topic, how you would have studied it, and what you expect to find.
- Read the authors' names and the abstract.
- Examine sources of funding, authors' employers, and authors' disclosures to discern possible author bias and/or conflict of interest.
- Identify terms and key concepts.
- Study the tables and graphs and read the results.
- Read the methods to determine whether the authors can justify their conclusions.
- Read the introduction and literature review and consider the significance, accuracy, appropriateness of studies, omissions, and thoroughness of explanations.
- Read the discussion and watch for speculation, suggestions for further research, and flaws or weaknesses.
- Read the results again to check that data is consistent with claims and that there is no other equal or better explanation.

LACTATION CONSULTANT PROFESSION

- Watch for spurious relationships.
- Determine what the researchers chose to include and exclude and why.

Leadership and Change

Effectiveness (From *The 7 Habits of Highly Effective People*, Stephen Covey, 1990).

- Choose to be effective: Choose your response and be proactive.
- Start with a blueprint: Plan before you act.
- Focus on what is important: Distinguish urgent from important, then prioritize, develop a timeline, and stay committed to your goals.
- Work toward mutual benefit: Create mutual benefits and focus on issues rather than on people.
- Understand other points of view: Attempt to see an issue from another person's point of view.
- Build a strong team: Work toward achieving unity and building a strong team.
- Take care of yourself: Be healthy physically and mentally with attention to exercise, nutrition, and stress.

The art of persuasion (Benjamin Franklin's acronym TALKING, Humes, 1992).

- ▶ **T**iming: Choose the right moment.
- ▶ **A**ppreciation: Appreciate the other person's problems and concerns.
- ▶ **L**istening: Listen well enough to find out what you need and how best to sell it.
- ▶ **K**nowledge: Learn the other person's viewpoint, and persuade them to see yours.
- ▶ **I**ntegrity: Maintain your fundamental beliefs or motives.
- ▶ **N**eed: Show them that they are uniquely qualified to give you what you need.
- ▶ **G**iving: Learn the value of giving.

Self-Confidence

- Approach every situation with the belief that you will succeed.
- Focus on the best way to do the job right and visualize yourself doing it.
- Trust in your ability to learn and use failure to build strength and wisdom.
- Be assertive when presenting your ideas to others.
- Learn how to resolve conflict.
  - Avoid confronting conflict in public or in the presence of others who are uninvolved.

Types of difficult people

▶ The aggressor is abrasive, abrupt, intimidating, and relentless—stay as dispassionate as possible, listen attentively, look them directly in the eye, and be ready to interrupt.

▶ The saboteur sabotages your efforts from behind the scene—expose their undermining efforts.

▶ The wet blanket dampens enthusiasm and undermines positive thinking—ask them for positive, realistic ways to solve problems and engage their talents.

▶ The expert may come across as pompous and arrogant and is usually very productive and talented—show that you respect their opinion, ask them to explain their point further, and be prepared and accurate in your interactions.

- Establish common goals, debate strategies, and find ways both can benefit by the outcome.
- Obtain support from others before a meeting and solicit their reactions when confronted.
- Use humor to diffuse conflict and resistance.

• Learn how to approach a difficult person.

- Give recognition and praise for accomplishments and avoid placing blame.
- Write down what you want to say to prepare for interactions.
- Face the person squarely, sit or stand erect, and lean forward.
- Give your undivided attention by responding verbally and nonverbally.
- Focus on the goal and what you are saying, and avoid distractions that could sidetrack you.
- Recycle the other person's message, and wait for a response before continuing to speak.

Change Agent

• Address a person's reasons for resisting change.

- Loss of control: Increase their involvement and participation, and empower them with legitimate choices and ownership.
- Uncertainty: Avoid springing decisions without groundwork or preparation.
- Difference: Minimize changes, and leave as many habits and routines unchanged as possible.
- Loss of face: Praise others for past accomplishments, and thank them for their willingness to change to meet present needs.
- Competence: Equip others with the knowledge and skills to perform under the new rules.

- Disruption: Support and recognize the extra energy, time, and mental pre-occupation.
- Past grievances: Address unresolved grievances that could color responses to the change.
- Real threat: Be sensitive to the loss of routines, comforts, traditions, and relationships.

• Facilitating change

- Do your homework: Collect as much supporting research and data as possible.
- Evaluate: Assess present policies and procedures, and identify those that can remain in place.
- Define the problem: Define specific areas that require change, and prepare detailed rationale.
- Define goals: Identify specific objectives for each proposed change.
- Anticipate: Write down anticipated arguments, possible responses, and other approaches.
- Prioritize: Start with the most acceptable changes to establish a record of accomplishment.
- Define strategies: Develop a time line for planning and implementing the change.
- Implement the change: Monitor responses for unanticipated problems and rectify them.
- Give recognition and praise: Recognize compliance with creative incentives or rewards.

• Form a diverse breastfeeding committee.

- Level of support: Include allies, resistors, and those who are neutral.
- Members: Consider members from obstetrics, labor and delivery, postpartum, neonatal intensive care, pediatrics, quality improvement, technicians, housekeeping, management, home care, pharmacy, speech pathology.

Seven stages of resistance to change (SARAR International):

▶ There is no problem. We don't need to change.

▶ I recognize there is a problem, but it's not my responsibility.

▶ I accept that there is a problem, but I doubt anyone's ability to change it.

▶ I accept that there is a problem, but I'm afraid to get involved.

▶ We have a problem, but I'm afraid to try to do anything about it.

▶ We know we can do it, and obstacles will not stop us.

▶ We did it, and now we want to share our results with others.

- Personality types: Include reactors, workaholics, rebels, persisters, dreamers, promoters, synthesists, idealists, pragmatists, analysts, and realists.

Promotion Efforts

- *International Code of Marketing of Breastmilk Substitutes* (see Appendix D)
- *Baby-friendly Hospital Initiative* (see Appendix E)
- *Global Strategy for Child and Young Infant Feeding*, WHO/UNICEF 2002

  - Develop comprehensive national policies on infant and young child feeding.
  - Use an evidence-based, integrated, comprehensive approach.
  - Consider the physical, social, economic, and cultural environment.
  - Support exclusive breastfeeding for 6 months in healthcare environments.
  - Increase exclusive breastfeeding rates in work environments.
  - Support breastfeeding with complementary foods up to 2 years and beyond.
  - Provide adequate, timely, safe complementary foods.
  - Guide families in exceptionally difficult circumstances.
  - Legislate and regulate adherence to the *International Code of Marketing of Breastmilk Substitutes*.

- National Breastfeeding Awareness Campaign (United States)

  - Encourage exclusive breastfeeding to 6 months of age.
  - Advertise the risks of *not* breastfeeding.

Tutorial for Students and Interns

Key Clinical Management Strategies

From *Clinical Guidelines for the Establishment of Exclusive Breastfeeding*, ILCA, 2005.

- Comply with the *International Code of Marketing of Breastmilk Substitutes*, and avoid distribution of infant feeding product samples and advertisements for such products.

Key Clinical Competencies

From *Clinical Competencies for IBCLC Practice* available at www.iblce.org.

☐ Conduct yourself in a professional manner, by complying with the profession's code of ethics, standards of practice, and the *International Code of Marketing of Breastmilk Substitutes* and its subsequent World Health Assembly resolutions.

LACTATION CONSULTANT PROFESSION

☐ Practice within the laws of the setting in which you work, showing respect for confidentiality and privacy.

☐ Advocate for breastfeeding families, mothers, infants and children in the workplace, community, and within the healthcare system.

☐ Demonstrate effective communication skills to maintain collaborative and supportive relationships.

☐ Make appropriate referrals to other healthcare professionals and community resources.

☐ Communicate effectively with other members of the healthcare team, using written documents appropriate to the location, facility and culture in which the student is being trained, such as consent forms, care plans, charting forms/clinical notes, pathways/care maps, and feeding assessment forms.

☐ Utilize current research findings to provide a strong evidence base for clinical practice, and obtain continuing education to enhance skills and obtain or maintain IBCLC certification.

☐ Use appropriate resources for research to provide information to the healthcare team on conditions and medications that affect breastfeeding and lactation.

☐ Use breastfeeding equipment appropriately and provide information about risks as well as benefits of products, maintaining an awareness of conflict of interest if profiting from the rental or sale of breastfeeding equipment.

☐ Obtain clinical experience in a lactation consultant private practice office.

☐ Obtain clinical experience in a private practice OB, pediatric, family practice, or midwifery office.

☐ Obtain clinical experience in a public health department; Women, Infants and Children (WIC) Program (in the United States).

☐ Obtain clinical experience in a hospital birthing center, postpartum unit, mother–baby unit, level II and level III nurseries (special care nursery and neonatal intensive care nursery), and pediatric unit.

☐ Obtain clinical experience in home health services.

☐ Obtain clinical experience in an outpatient follow-up breastfeeding clinic.

☐ Obtain clinical experience with home birth (if legally permitted).

☐ Obtain clinical experience in a volunteer community support group meeting.

From Theory to Practice

1. The elements of a lactation management program presented in this text are the areas covered by the grid for the certification exam. Which areas are your strengths and which are your weaknesses? How will you address the areas of weakness?

2. How will you arrange obtaining supervised clinical experience?

3. Where are you along the spectrum of acquiring the role of lactation consultant?

4. What are the dangers in failing to proceed beyond the formal stage of role acquisition?

5. What will be the nature of your role with mothers when you are at the informal stage of acquiring the role of lactation consultant?
6. What are your goals after you reach the personal stage of role acquisition?
7. How do ethics influence behavior?
8. What are the elements of living an ethical life?
9. Why is it difficult to be ethical all the time?
10. What guides your ethical practice as a lactation consultant?
11. Considering all the possible practice settings for a lactation consultant, what are the advantages and disadvantages of each setting?
12. How will you know if you are starting to feel burned out as a lactation consultant?
13. How can you prevent becoming burned out?
14. Which of the pitfalls in counseling are you most at risk for experiencing? How can you avoid them?
15. Which type of research article would be least likely to form an appropriate basis for changing practices? Why?
16. What helpful insights might you gather from learning the names of research study's authors?
17. What can you learn about the validity of research findings by knowing the methods used in the study?
18. Why is it not a good idea to rely on only reading the results and discussion of a research article?
19. Which of the study designs do you consider the most valid? Why?
20. What is the significance of an unbalanced bell curve?
21. Which of the tests used in a study provide information about statistical significance?
22. What kinds of questions might you ask yourself after you read the discussion portion of a research article?
23. What kinds of questions might you ask yourself after you read the results portion of a research article?
24. How might the sources of funding or author relationships with industry affect the study's findings and presentation of those findings?
25. Stephen Covey wrote *The 7 Habits of Highly Effective People*. Which of the habits do you think will help you become a more effective person?
26. How can you become more confident in your interactions with others?
27. Which of the seven stages of resistance to change do you consider the most difficult in your interactions with colleagues?
28. You spent over an hour working with a mother to help her with effective positioning and latch. You checked back with her for the next two feedings and found her using ineffective techniques both times. How will you respond, and what will be your first statement to her?
29. You set up a pumping routine for the mother of a premature infant yet each time you check with her she indicates she is not pumping very often. How will you respond, and what will be your first statement to her?

30. One of the mothers from your breastfeeding class called you several times in the weeks before she delivered. Her enthusiasm for breastfeeding was infectious, and you enjoyed sharing in her anticipation. Her baby was born with galactosemia, making it impossible to breastfeed. She is despondent over the loss of her plans to breastfeed. How will you respond, and what will be your first statement to her? How will you deal with your own disappointment?

31. One of the physicians in your community continually advises mothers to supplement their babies with formula if the baby is greater than 7% below birth weight at 2 days postpartum. It occurred with a mother you visited on rounds today. How will you respond, and what will be your first statement to the mother? How will you deal with your frustration?

32. Your breastfeeding committee has been working toward making your hospital baby-friendly. There has been a great deal of resistance from a vocal group of nurses who seem to sabotage every effort. Considering the material presented on creating change, develop a plan for addressing this problem. In your plan, address stages of resistance, reasons for resistance, conflict resolution, the art of persuasion, elements in facilitating change, and the makeup of the committee.

CHAPTER 4

Clinical
Practice

In This Chapter

Documents that Guide Professional Practice

Standards of Practice

- Standards promote consistency by encouraging a common, systematic approach.
- Standards are specific in content to guide daily practice.
- Standards provide a framework for policies, protocols, educational programs, and quality improvement efforts.
- Standards apply to diverse practice settings and cultural contexts.
- See Appendix B for *Standards of Practice for International Board Certified Lactation Consultants.*

The International Code of Marketing of Breastmilk Substitutes

- The World Health Assembly created the *Code* in 1981.
- The *Code* calls for regulating marketing and distribution of products that replace human milk.
- Several subsequent resolutions supplement and further promote the *Code.*
- See Appendix D for main provisions of the *Code.*

Clinical Competencies

- Competencies identify the skills needed to provide safe and effective care.
- Competencies include situations and challenges encountered most frequently.

- See competencies from *Clinical Competencies for IBCLC Practice* at the end of each chapter. Complete document is available at www.iblce.org.

Clinical Guidelines

- Clinical guidelines provide an operational framework for optimal breastfeeding management.
- Clinical guidelines address common problems, circumstances, and conditions that may require referral to an IBCLC.
- See clinical guidelines from *Clinical Guidelines for the Establishment of Exclusive Breastfeeding* at the end of each chapter. Complete document is available at www.ilca.org.

Elements of a Consultation

Consent

- Obtain signed consent, if necessary, before initiating a consultation.
- Elements of a consent form:

  - Work with the mother and infant at this and all subsequent visits.
  - Examine the mother's breasts and nipples.
  - Perform an examination of the infant including a digital oral examination.
  - Observe a breastfeeding.
  - Demonstrate or use equipment and techniques that will improve breastfeeding.
  - Release information to the insurance company.
  - Send reports to the primary caregivers and consult with them regarding their care.
  - Use information obtained from the consultation for educational purposes.
  - Take photographs for educational use.
  - Receive payment for the consultation and rental or sale of breastfeeding equipment.
  - Comply with privacy requirements (Health Insurance Portability and Accountability Act in the United States).

History

- Use guiding skills to gather information and impressions.
- Elements of a history:

  - Health of the mother and infant, past and present
  - The mother's perception of any problem and when it began
  - History of previous breastfeeding and details about current breastfeeding
  - Medications taken by the mother and baby, past and present

- The baby's feeding and growth patterns, sleeping, crying, and ability to socialize
- Patterns of stooling and voiding, and amounts in the last 24-hour period

Assessment

- Assess the baby, the mother, the mother's breasts, and breastfeeding (see Chapter 6 for detailed assessments).
- Observations to note and record:

  - Interactions between the mother and baby
  - Dynamics of the feeding process
  - The baby's oral and facial structure
  - The baby's and mother's temperaments, behavior, and emotional status
  - Appearance and condition of the mother's breasts and nipples
  - Evidence of milk transfer
  - The mother's economic and employment status
  - The mother's support network and cultural beliefs and practices
  - The mother's breastfeeding goals

Plan of Care

- Empower the mother and increase her self-confidence and self-reliance.

  - Actively involve her in developing a plan of care.
  - Determine what she needs to know.
  - Have a clear and specific purpose for any intervention.

- Begin with essentials of feeding the baby, the mother's pain relief, and milk production.

  - Help her understand what produced her situation and how she can avoid its recurrence.
  - Suggest options and be mindful of her reactions.
  - Ask her to repeat the plan, and summarize it with her to avoid confusion.

- Provide the mother with necessary resources.

  - Give her a written plan of care.
  - Refer her to a community support group.

Follow-Up

- Arrange follow-up with the mother as appropriate.
- Send a report to caregivers as appropriate (see Figure 4-1).
- Evaluate the consultation (see Figure 4-2).
- Review your counseling skills (see Figure 4-3).

Elements of a Physician Report

1. Date the patient was seen
2. Names and addresses of mother's physician and baby's physician
3. Regarding: Mother's and baby's names and baby's date of birth
4. Dear Dr. . . . ,
5. Patient was seen at your request, was self-referred, was referred by (include name if possible)
6. If you called the physician's office to give a verbal report or faxed in a short report, you can mention this in your letter.
7. Because of . . . (reason for referral)
8. Brief description of the mother's history (general health, conception, pregnancy, and birth)
9. Assessment of the mother's breasts and nipples
10. Brief description of the baby's history (birth, Apgar scores, in-hospital feeding, current feedings, output, weights, behavior, etc.)
11. Assessment and present status of the baby (muscle tone, activity, skin turgor, oral cavity, behavior, weight, and so on)
12. Assessment of the feeding (include feeding weights, if possible)
13. Your assessment of the situation
14. Suggestions you made to the mother and the action plan that was developed
15. Arrangements for follow-up with the mother
16. If the patient was referred to you, thank the physician for allowing you to participate in the care of the patient. If the patient was self-referred, you may comment about working with the physician with this couple ("It was a pleasure . . .").
17. Sincerely yours, . . . (use your credentials behind your name)

Figure 4-1 Elements of a Physician Report

Documentation

- Document every contact.
- Teach mothers to chart their information.
- Use a standard documentation method for all staff (see Appendix F).

  - Breastfeed observation form
  - Breastfeeding descriptors
  - The LATCH method
  - The mother–baby assessment method (MBA)
  - The infant breastfeeding assessment tool (IBFAT)

Questions to Measure the Quality of a Consultation

1. My confidence in my counseling skills has increased over the past 6 months.
2. I have identified the counseling style in which I am most comfortable and effective.
3. I am able to adapt my counseling style to meet the needs of the patient.
4. I am now using more attending and listening skills in my counseling sessions.
5. I am now able to recognize when a patient is not attending or listening during the counseling process.
6. I am better able to acknowledge my feelings that arise during the counseling process.
7. I am better able to acknowledge the feelings of my patients during the counseling process.
8. I have altered the way I conduct the counseling session based on the recognition of my own or my patient's feelings.
9. I evaluate the counseling environment before beginning the counseling session.
10. I take steps to correct the environment before beginning the counseling session.
11. I have requested that management make changes in my work site counseling environment that will enhance the counseling process.
12. I need further instruction, encouragement, or evaluation to enhance my counseling skills.

Figure 4-2 Questions to Measure the Quality of a Consultation

---

Questions to Evaluate Counseling Skills in a Consultation

1. Understanding of the problem: Consultant understood the mother and helped her.
2. Breastfeeding information: Information was correct and appropriate. Not too much or too little.
3. Clarity of instructions: The mother understood the information and advice.
4. Good counseling skills: Consultant put mother at ease, encouraged her to share feelings.
5. Partnership with mother: Mother was drawn into the problem-solving process.
6. Encouraged mother's self-reliance: Consultant fostered greater self-assurance in mother.
7. Balance: Consultant achieved balance between listening, educating, and problem solving with no lecturing.
8. Arrangements for follow-up: Consultant made it clear when any further contact will take place and who will initiate it.
9. Overall impressions of mother's satisfaction with consultation.

Figure 4-3 Questions to Evaluate Counseling Skills in a Consultation

Tutorial for Students and Interns

Key Clinical Competencies
From *Clinical Competencies for IBCLC Practice* available at www.iblce.org.

- ☐ Obtain the mother's permission for providing care to her or her baby.
- ☐ Obtain a pertinent history.
- ☐ Communicate effectively with other members of the healthcare team, using written documents appropriate to the location, facility, and culture in which the student is being trained, such as: consent forms, care plans, charting forms/clinical notes, pathways/care maps, and feeding assessment forms.
- ☐ Write referrals and follow-up documentation or letters to referring and primary healthcare providers.
- ☐ Make appropriate referrals to other healthcare professionals and community resources.

From Theory to Practice
Clinical Competencies and Guidelines

1. How can you enhance your communication and counseling skills with mothers?
2. How can you ensure that you obtain a complete and useful history of a mother and baby?
3. What are the important elements to include in an infant assessment?
4. How can you routinely share information with physicians about the mothers and babies in your care?
5. What sort of information do you need to share with physicians about the mothers and babies in your care?
6. How can you ensure that a mother receives appropriate teaching and assistance in the first 2 hours after birth?
7. How can you share all of the information indicated under postpartum skills without overwhelming the mother?
8. How can you incorporate a mother in problem solving and developing a plan of care?
9. Which maternal and infant breastfeeding challenges are not typically encountered in your usual practice setting? How and where can you acquire competency in those areas?
10. When is it appropriate to assess milk transfer with the use of pre- and post-feed weights?
11. Which technology and devices are appropriate to teach to every mother, and which should be reserved for special situations?
12. How can you ensure that your knowledge base is current regarding the various techniques and devices?

13. How and where can you acquire competency in the breastfeeding challenges that are encountered infrequently?
14. Why is it useful to acquire clinical skills in a variety of settings?
15. How can you use the *Clinical Guidelines for the Establishment of Exclusive Breastfeeding* to achieve consistency in advice given to mothers?

Standards of Practice

16. How do the ILCA *Standards of Practice* guide the day-to-day performance of a lactation consultant?
17. Which members of the healthcare profession should practice within the lactation consultant profession's standards of practice?
18. How can you ensure that you consistently obtain and document necessary information for a mother and baby? Why is this important?
19. How can you ensure that you provide appropriate follow-up and reporting of a consultation?
20. What kinds of outcomes might cause you to modify a mother's plan of care?
21. What anticipatory teaching will increase a mother's self-confidence?
22. How can you ensure that you are providing appropriate emotional support to the mothers in your care?
23. What obstacles or challenges do you face in adhering to the *International Code of Marketing of Breastmilk Substitutes*?
24. What is your personal code on the use of breastfeeding equipment and devices?
25. How can you arrange to have your clinical practices evaluated?
26. How do you ensure that your clinical practice is research based?
27. How can you determine if a mother understood the plan of care?
28. What situations might require a mother and baby to be seen rather than helped over the telephone?
29. In your own personal circumstances, what particular situations would you refer to another lactation consultant or healthcare provider?

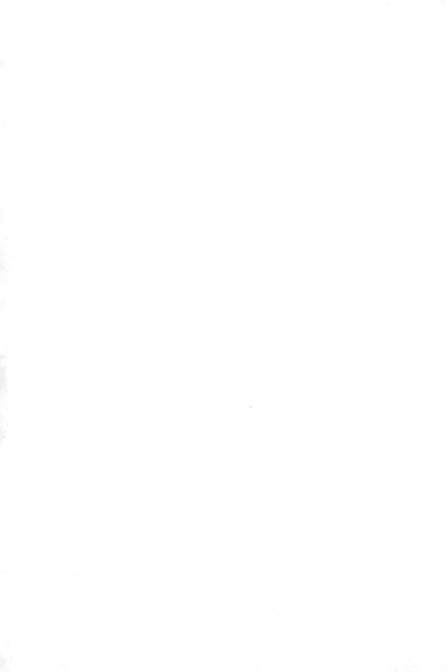

CHAPTER 5

Science of Lactation

In This Chapter

Breast Anatomy

External Features

- Skin layers:

  - The **dermis** (inner layer) contains nerve endings, capillaries, hair follicles, lymph channels, and other cells.
  - The **epidermis** (outer layer) contains epithelial cells that cover and protect deeper skin layers from drying out and from invasion by bacteria.
  - The **germinating layer** (transitional layer) contains basal cells that continually divide. New cells constantly push older ones up toward the surface of the skin.
  - **Keratin** (the surface layer) contains tough, protective protein. It is dead skin.

- Nipple:

  - There are about 7 to 10 nipple duct openings.

    ‣ **Smooth muscle fibers** function as a closing mechanism for the milk ducts.
    ‣ **Sensory nerve endings** in the nipple trigger milk release when the baby suckles.

- An inverted nipple appears inverted or inverts when stimulated.

  - ▶ It will respond to correction during the last trimester of pregnancy.
  - ▶ Women at risk for premature labor should not stimulate their nipples.
  - ▶ With a large portion of the breast in the baby's mouth inversion usually is not a problem.

- Areola:

  - The areola enlarges and becomes darker during puberty, menstruation, and pregnancy.
  - The baby's mouth needs to enclose a large portion to compress sufficient breast tissue.

- Montgomery glands (Montgomery's tubercles):

  - Sebaceous glands are located around the areola and are pimply in appearance.
  - They secrete an oily substance to lubricate and protect the nipple.
  - They are rudimentary mammary glands and may secrete a small amount of milk.

Internal Features

- Connective tissues support the breast and subcutaneous fatty tissues give it shape.

  - Fibrous bands (**Cooper's ligaments**) support the breast.
  - Fibrous tissue holds the breast together and supports the ducts as they fill with milk.

- Nerves trigger milk synthesis and release.

  - Sensory fibers innervate smooth muscle in the nipple and blood vessels from the fourth, fifth, and sixth intercostal nerves.
  - The nipple and areola are composed of autonomic and sensory nerves.
  - The epidermis of the nipple and areola has few nerves.
  - The dermis is highly innervated and responsive to suckling stimulation.

- Blood and lymph systems:

  - The bloodstream transports proteins, fats, carbohydrates, and other substances to the cells for milk production.
  - The lymphatic system absorbs excess blood fluids and returns them to the heart.
  - Lymph nodes filter and trap bacteria and cast-off cell parts.
  - Swelling of a lymph node in the armpit could suggest an infection in the breast, arm, or hand.
  - Engorgement decreases the flow of blood and lymph, increasing the risk of local infection.

- Fatty tissue:

  - There is very little fat immediately beneath the areola and nipple.
  - Fatty tissue does not contribute to milk synthesis or transport.
  - Women with larger breasts may be more likely to have a larger storage capacity, though size is not a predictor of production.

- Glandular tissue is the functional part of the breast that produces and transports milk.

  - Milk production takes place in tiny individual glands called **alveoli** or acini.

    - Alveoli consist of epithelial cells (lactocytes) encased by myoepithelial cells and are clustered together to form lobuli.
    - Capillaries surrounding the alveoli bring nutrient-rich blood to make milk.
    - Release of oxytocin and prolactin signal myoepithelial cells to contract the alveoli to release and produce more milk.
    - The normal lactating breast is lumpy due to enlarged milk-filled alveoli.
    - Alveoli multiply and increase in size during pregnancy and lactation, then decrease in size and number when breastfeeding ends.

  - The **tail of Spence** is breast tissue that extends into the axilla.

- Milk-transporting tissue (see Figure 5-1):

  - Milk flows through a system of lactiferous ductules, secondary ducts, and nipple pores.
  - Ducts grow lengthwise as alveoli and lobuli develop.
  - Sprouting and growth of ducts and alveolar development intensify during the first 4 to 5 months of pregnancy.
  - Duct and alveolar tissues become more specialized in the second half of pregnancy in preparation for milk-related functions.
  - Ducts widen throughout the breast and in the area beneath the areola during passage of milk.

SCIENCE OF LACTATION

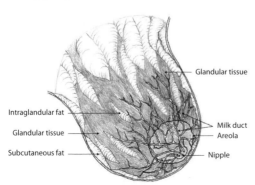

Figure 5-1
Anatomy of the Breast.
Source: Geddes DT, Hartmann RL, Hartmann PE. University of Western Australia's Human Lactation Research Group. Printed with permission.

Breast Anomalies

- Differences in physical features:

  - A **galactocele** is a cyst caused by obstruction of one or more mammary ducts. It may resolve spontaneously or it can be compressed, aspirated, or removed surgically.
  - An **intraductal papilloma** is a small benign growth in a milk duct that produces a bloody discharge.
  - **Paget's disease** is a cancerous condition that produces scaly, itchy nipples and areolas and sometimes a bloody discharge.
  - **Hypoplasia** is widely spaced, tubular and thin breasts, a marker for insufficient glandular tissue.

- Signs of possible glandular insufficiency:

  - There is no noticeable change in breast size during pregnancy or lactation.
  - One breast is appreciably smaller than the other breast.
  - There is a family history of lactation failure.
  - Milk production is inadequate despite appropriate feeding practices.
  - **Ductal atresia** (lack of a milk duct opening) prevents milk secretion from that duct.

- Evidence of surgery:

  - Women with a history of breast surgery may still have functional tissue.

    - Breast augmentation may damage nerves but usually does not destroy functional tissue.
    - Breast reduction is more intrusive and often affects lactation.
    - Resection of the nipple severs all ducts and usually prevents a full milk supply.
    - The pedicle technique transposes the nipple, areola, and ducts. Breastfeeding may be possible if the nerve supply to the breast remains intact.
    - Women previously treated for breast cancer who do not show any evidence of a residual tumor can breastfeed.
    - Breast, chest, back, or cardiac surgery can affect blood flow and innervation to the nipple.

  - A mother can attempt to breastfeed and monitor her baby's output and weight.
  - Milk production may respond to galactogogues, external oxytocin, or increased stimulation.
  - Provide early and frequent follow-up for evaluation of feeding effectiveness.

Breast Physiology

Breast Development and Milk Synthesis

- Puberty and pregnancy are the times of most functional breast tissue development.

    - Increased estrogen during menstruation produces the growth of ducts and connective tissue.
    - In the absence of pregnancy, tissue growth regresses and glandular cells degenerate.
    - Breast development is far more significant during pregnancy than during menstruation.

- **Mammogenesis** occurs during the first trimester of pregnancy.

    - The duct system multiplies and the skin stretches to accommodate internal enlargement.
    - The nipple and areola increase in circumference.
    - The areola darkens and the Montgomery glands become noticeable.

- Colostrum production begins during the second trimester.
- **Stage I lactogenesis** occurs during the third trimester.

    - The breast begins to gather the nutrients needed for milk synthesis.
    - Lactose, total proteins, and immunoglobulins increase.
    - Sodium and chloride decrease.

- **Stage II lactogenesis** occurs at around day 2 to 5 postpartum.

    - Blood flow within the breast increases.
    - Transitional milk production and copious milk secretion begin.

- **Stage III lactogenesis** (galactopoiesis) occurs at around day 8 to 10 postpartum.

    - Establishment and maintenance of mature milk occurs.
    - Milk production continues until weaning.

- **Involution** occurs after weaning and the breast slowly returns to its prepregnant state.

Hormonal Control

- Several hormones are involved in milk production.

    - **Estrogen** stimulates growth of the uterus, vagina, and other reproductive organs.
    - **Progesterone** inhibits prolactin's effects during pregnancy.
    - **Prolactin** stimulates alveolar growth and milk synthesis, and induces maternal behavior.

- Unlimited, effective suckling during the night maintains high prolactin levels.
- **Oxytocin** releases in response to suckling and contracts the myoepithelial cells to eject milk.

- Hormones respond to the frequency and degree of breast drainage.

  - Frequent feeding increases prolactin levels by increasing prolactin receptors.
  - The **prolactin inhibitory factor** (PIF) prevents prolactin release when the baby is not suckling. Suckling inhibits the PIF to allow prolactin release.
  - Autocrine control through the human whey protein, **feedback inhibitor of lactation** (FIL), inhibits milk synthesis when milk remains in the breast.

Milk Ejection Reflex (Letdown)

- Suckling stimulates nerve endings and sends a message to the hypothalamus.

  - The message goes to the anterior pituitary, lowers the PIF and triggers prolactin release.
  - The posterior pituitary gland secretes oxytocin and contracts alveoli and uterus muscles.
  - The contraction forces milk down through the lactiferous duct system to the nipple.

- Letdown moves fat globules down through the ducts (hindmilk) to provide higher calorie milk.
- Fatigue, anxiety, fear, pain, or weak stimulation from ineffective latch can inhibit letdown.
- Signs of letdown:

  - Milk drips from one breast while the baby is nursing on the other breast.
  - The mother may feel fullness, tingling, or a burning sensation in her breasts.
  - The mother experiences increased thirst or sleepiness.
  - The mother experiences uterine contractions in the early days postpartum.
  - The baby begins gulping or gagging from the sudden rush of milk.
  - The mother hears more pronounced swallowing.

Hormonal Anomalies

- Pituitary, thyroid, and adrenal imbalances can affect milk production and release.
- **Sheehan's syndrome** (hypopituitarism) resulting from severe postpartum hemorrhage and hypotension can cause irreversible damage to milk-producing cells.

> **ADVICE TO CLINICIANS**
> **TEACH MOTHERS**
> ▶ How to preserve the keratin layer and lubrication of skin on the nipple
> ▶ To take in about a 1-inch diameter of areolar tissue
> ▶ That the baby needs to grasp the breast well and suckle vigorously to stimulate the deeper nerves
> ▶ That breast size corresponds to fatty and glandular tissue and not to milk synthesis or transport
> ▶ That breast sagging is a result of pregnancy, not lactation
> ▶ That suckling signals more blood to provide the nutrients needed to make milk
> ▶ That engorgement decreases the flow of blood and lymph, causes edema, increases the risk of local infection, and leads to poor milk drainage
> ▶ That frequent feedings, good positioning at the breast, and pumping in the absence of effective and frequent suckling will protect milk production

SCIENCE OF LACTATION

- **Polycystic ovarian syndrome** (Stein-Leventhal syndrome) is associated with insufficient milk supply.
- A **prolactinoma** is not a reason for a mother to not breastfeed.
- Thyroid supplementation for hypothyroidism does not compromise the baby's health.

Physiology of Milk Transfer

Sucking

- The baby draws the breast into his mouth and maintains negative pressure to keep it there.
- **Nonnutritive sucking** has low flow with a light suck, almost a flutter.

  - There are short jaw excursions and little or no audible swallowing.
  - It elicits about two sucks per second.
  - It indicates the baby is trying to make milk available.

- **Nutritive sucking** has high flow with a long, deep suck–swallow–breathe pattern.

  - It elicits about one suck per second.
  - It is affected by central nervous system (CNS) depressants.
  - It indicates effective milk transfer.

Effects of Sucking

- Effects on the baby:

  - Sucking is a means of comfort and nourishment.
  - Sucking stimulates saliva, gastrointestinal secretions, hormones, and motility, helping the baby pass gas and stool.
  - Sucking releases the hormone **cholecystokinin** (CCK) to promote satiety and sleepiness.
  - A baby's need for sucking is usually greatest in the first 3 months.

- Effects on the mother:

  - Prolactin release stimulates milk production and maternal yearning.
  - Oxytocin release causes cuddly and warm feelings, triggers milk to let down, and contracts the uterus.

Sucking Pattern

- Sucking rhythm corresponds inversely to the amount of milk available.

  - Sucking alternates between nutritive and nonnutritive sucking throughout the feeding.
  - The baby adjusts the sucking rate to cope with letdown.
  - Sucking is rapid at the beginning of a feeding to initiate milk flow.
  - Sucking pace slows when letdown occurs and the baby swallows.
  - Rapid sucking resumes, stimulates further milk flow, and then slows as milk flows.

- Nutritive sucking has a regular rhythm of suck–swallow–breathe.

  - Swallowing cannot occur simultaneously with breathing.
  - The baby pauses between bursts of sucking and regulates breathing.

    - On days 2–3, the mother has a small volume of colostrum, and the baby sucks with several short, fast bursts per swallow.
    - On days 3–4, the mother is producing transitional milk with increased volume and the baby establishes a regular rhythm.
    - On days 4–5, milk flows following letdown and the baby swallows with every suck.

  - Preterm infants have fewer sucks per burst and longer pauses. They can coordinate suck–swallow–breathing as easily when breastfeeding as when bottle feeding.

Suckling

- The baby suckles milk from the breast with tongue compression.

    - The baby's tongue draws the nipple and areola into his mouth.
    - A cone-shaped extension of the breast conforms to the shape of the baby's mouth.
    - The areola and nipple press upward progressively against the upper gum, hard palate, and soft palate.
    - The gums alternately compress and release as milk flows.

- Consequences of ineffective suckling:

    - The mother is at risk for engorgement, plugged ducts, mastitis, and compromised milk production.
    - The baby is at risk for increased hunger, fussiness, coliclike symptoms, low urine and stool output, jaundice, and inadequate weight gain or weight loss.

- Causes of disorganized suckling:

    - Illness or prematurity
    - Drugs given to the infant or mother
    - Delay in the first breastfeeding at birth
    - Neuromotor dysfunction
    - Variations in oral anatomy
    - Nipple preference due to artificial nipple use
    - Vigorous oral suctioning at birth
    - Birth trauma such as forceps, vacuum, or bruising

Milk Transfer

- Milk transfer requires a functioning letdown, appropriate suckling, and an effective latch.
- The transfer process:

    - The baby draws the end of the nipple back almost to the soft palate.
    - The front tip of the tongue wells up and the lower jaw rises.
    - The jaws compress the breast and pinch off milk in the lactiferous ducts.
    - The tongue pushes against the hard palate and compresses the lactiferous ducts.
    - When the baby's jaw opens, more milk is released from the breast.
    - Milk reaches the back of the baby's mouth and stimulates the baby to swallow.
    - The back of the tongue depresses to create negative pressure and maintain latch.

SCIENCE OF LACTATION

- Differences between milk transfer in breastfeeding and bottle feeding

  - The baby combines sucking and suckling in breastfeeding:

    ‣ The baby's lips, gums, tongue, cheeks, and hard and soft palate mold the breast to the size and shape of the baby's mouth.
    ‣ The baby actively suckles to receive milk.

  - The baby sucks in bottle feeding:

    ‣ The baby draws in the nipple and must alter the shape of the mouth to accommodate the shape of the artificial nipple.
    ‣ The baby must generate suction pressure so milk flows freely from the bottle.
    ‣ To control flow, the baby may thrust his tongue against the nipple. This motion may transfer to breastfeeding and create problems.

Human Milk
Properties of Human Milk

- Colostrum is the first milk.

  - Residual materials in the breast mix with newly formed milk.
  - Colostrum is richer than mature milk in sodium, potassium, chloride, protein, fat-soluble vitamins, and minerals.
  - Colostrum contains less fat and lactose than mature milk.
  - Colostrum has high concentrations of IgA, IgG and IgM (higher than mature milk).
  - Colostrum engulfs and digests disease organisms and aids in rapid gut closure.

- Fat content varies from mother to mother and from feeding to feeding.

  - Fat is inversely proportional to the time between feedings and the degree of breast fullness.
  - Fat may be up to 4 to 5 times higher at the end of a feeding.
  - Fat decreases in the later months of lactation.
  - Long-chain polyunsaturated fatty acids promote optimal neural and visual development.

- Composition and volume are variable.

  - Milk is high in immunoglobulins and protein during the first several weeks.
  - Volume is dependent on regular removal of milk.
  - Human milk can provide 75% of nutrient needs from about 8 months through 12 months of age.
  - Daily output during the second year is typically about 8 ounces.

- Lactose, lactase and lipase:

  - **Lactose** is the most constant among mothers of all the constituents in human milk.

    ‣ Lactose enhances calcium absorption and prevents rickets.
    ‣ Lactose supplies energy to the brain and is essential to central nervous system development.
    ‣ Lactose protects the intestine from the growth of harmful organisms.

  - **Lactase** converts lactose into simple sugars that the infant can absorb.
  - Lactase and **lipase** protect babies born with immature or defective enzyme systems.
  - A deficiency in lactase can result in lactose intolerance.

- Digestive properties protect the infant.

  - The **curd** is soft, small, less compact and easier to digest than artificial baby milk.
  - **Oligosaccharides** prevent pathogens from binding to receptor sites in the gut.
  - **IgA** protects the GI tract and is the most important of the antiviral defense factors.
  - **Bifidus factor** works with the pH of the stool to discourage the growth of *E. coli*.
  - **Lactoferrin** inhibits the growth of *E. coli*; its effects decrease if saturated with exogenous iron.
  - **Lysozyme** breaks down bacteria in the bowel and protects against Enterobacteriaceae and gram-positive bacteria.
  - **Alpha-lactalbumin** inhibits bacteria and yeast growth.
  - **Xantine oxidase** combined with nitrites inhibits *E. coli* and *Salmonella enteritidis*.
  - **Nucleotides** promote optimal function and growth of the GI and immune systems.

- Other properties:

  - High levels of antibodies protect the lining of the infant's intestine from absorption and enhance infant antibody response.
  - Protein is relatively constant regardless of the mother's diet.
  - All vitamins are sufficient, with sun exposure for additional vitamin D.
  - Healthy nonanemic mothers lay down sufficient iron stores for the first few months.
  - Suckling triggers cholecystokinin (CCK) and causes sleepiness in mothers and babies.
  - Mucins in human milk protect against bacterial infections.
  - Thyroid hormones prevent hypothyroidism, mask diagnosis, and protect the baby until weaning.

SCIENCE OF LACTATION

- Properties of milk of women who deliver prematurely:

  - The milk is higher in sodium, chloride, nitrogen, and immunoprotective factors.
  - **Human milk fortifiers** (HMF)—protein, calcium, potassium phosphate, carbohydrates, vitamins and trace minerals—are used to supplement infants with very low birth weights.
  - **Lactoengineering offers** an alternative to HMF by isolating hindmilk to increase calories, carbohydrates, and proteins for preterm infants.

Health Benefits of Human Milk

- The child has fewer dental caries and better dental health.
- Benefits are dose-dependent in increasing IQ.
- The child receives lifelong protection against upper and lower respiratory infections, otitis media, diarrheal disease, urinary tract infections, sepsis, rotavirus, meningitis, leukemia, lymphoma, Hodgkin's disease, and neuroblastoma.
- There is a lower risk of necrotizing enterocolitis (NEC), asthma, breast cancer, chronic and autoimmune diseases, hypertension, high cholesterol, and heart disease.
- Bacteria are destroyed in the GI tract before they affect the infant.
- Antibodies are produced to fight against organisms that pass into the breast from the suckling infant.
- Maternal antigens to a cold, fever, or more serious illness protect her breast-fed baby.

Storage and Use of Expressed Milk

- Collection and storage guidelines (see Figure 5-2):

Storage Recommendations		
Temperature	**Healthy baby**	**Baby in the NICU**
Room temperature	Up to 6 hours	Up to 4 hours
Insulated cooler with gel paks	Up to 24 hours	Up to 24 hours
Refrigerator	Up to 8 days	Up to 8 days
Refrigerator freezer	Up to 6 months	Up to 3 months
Deep freezer	Up to 12 months	Up to 6 months

Figure 5-2 Storage Recommendations.
Source: Human Milk Banking Association of North America

- Glass or hard plastic are preferred for storage; soft plastic reduces antibodies in milk.
- Store in amounts the baby will consume, leaving room for expansion.
- Label and use the oldest milk first.
- Chill newly pumped milk before adding it to refrigerated or frozen milk.
- Freeze milk if it will not be used within 3 to 8 days.
- Frozen milk with a bad odor may be due to lipase levels; warm the milk to scalding and immediately freeze to prevent this.

- Defrosting and warming milk:

  - Thawed milk may remain refrigerated for up to 24 hours before use.
  - Place frozen milk in a refrigerator overnight for a slow thaw.
  - Thaw frozen milk rapidly in a pan of warm water or under a stream of warm tap water.
  - Do not use a microwave oven to warm milk.
  - Milk that has been warmed must be used immediately and only for that feeding.
  - Do not refreeze milk.

- Guidelines for the neonatal intensive care unit (NICU):

  - Express milk just before feeding it to the baby.
  - If the baby will not receive the milk within one hour, refrigerate it immediately.
  - Place the milk from each pumping session in a separate container to minimize handling.
  - Talk with the NICU staff regarding how much to store for feedings to avoid waste.

Safety of Human Milk

- Medications:

  - Most medications are compatible with breastfeeding.
  - In general, a relative infant dose of less than 10% is considered safe.
  - Use drug information from well-documented sources.
  - Become acquainted with drug groups and their risks and benefits.
  - Questions to ask about a particular medication:

    ‣ Will it pass into the mother's milk and be absorbed in the baby's GI tract?
    ‣ Can the baby safely be exposed to the substance as it appears in the milk?
    ‣ How soon after birth will it be taken?
    ‣ What is the baby's gestational age?
    ‣ How resistant is it to detoxification?

- Mothers can minimize the effects of a medication.

    ▹ Take it immediately after nursing or 3 to 4 hours before the next feeding.
    ▹ Avoid nursing when it is at its peak level in the milk.
    ▹ Avoid drugs with a long half-life.
    ▹ Select the least offensive drug.

- Social toxicants:

    ▪ Newborn and preterm babies are susceptible to caffeine because it takes time to eliminate.
    ▪ Generally, an occasional drink socially is not a problem.
    ▪ A mother may breastfeed when the effects of alcohol have worn off.
    ▪ Reduce or eliminate smoking, as toxins do go to the infant and may increase irritability and the risk of SIDS. If necessary to continue, smoke outside and after breastfeeding.

- Environmental contaminants:

    ▪ Silicone breast implants have not been proven dangerous in breastfeeding.
    ▪ Toxins are primarily deposited in fat and are excreted in the mother's milk.
    ▪ Flame-retardant chemicals affect learning, memory, behavior, thyroid hormones, and other bodily functions.
    ▪ PCBs affect mental development.
    ▪ DDE affects protection against atopic disorders such as asthma, eczema, and hay fever.

ADVICE TO CLINICIANS

TEACH MOTHERS

▸ Consider alternatives that do not involve medication or substitute a safer medication.

▸ Weigh benefits of a medication against possible risk to the baby.

▸ Weigh the risk of a medication to the baby against the risk of artificial baby milk.

▸ Avoid nicotine and tobacco or time breastfeeding to minimize exposure in the milk.

▸ Avoid excessive alcohol consumption.

▸ Avoid all drugs of abuse.

▸ Avoid occupations, hobbies, and clothes that involve possible exposure to chemicals.

▸ Avoid eating shark, swordfish, king mackerel, and tilefish.

▸ Limit consumption of canned albacore tuna and other fish.

▸ Avoid eating organ meats.

▸ Wash or peel fresh fruits and vegetables.

Artificial Baby Milk

Artificial Baby Milk (ABM) Is Inferior to Human Milk

- Each brand is only slightly different yet all are intended to meet universal needs of infants.
- They are deficient in many constituents essential for optimum infant growth and health.
- Some have excessive or deficient amounts of micronutrients or macronutrients.
- Some completely lack essential elements.
- Some have lower levels of nervonic acid (NA), docosapentaenoic (DPA) acid, and DHA.
- Some have excessive vitamin D, which is toxic in high doses.
- Some are deficient in chloride.

Legitimate need for a baby to receive ABM:

▶ Conditions in the mother:
  - Sheehan's syndrome
  - Long-term drug therapy
  - Severe congestive heart failure
  - Insufficient milk supply
  - Tuberculosis (until after treatment)
  - HIV
  - Active herpes lesion
  - Eclampsia
  - Cytotoxic or radioactive drugs
▶ Conditions in the baby:
  - Galactosemia
  - Hypoglycemia or dehydration if unimproved by increased breastfeeding and no human milk is available
  - Prematurity if no human milk is available—use of human milk fortifier with VLBW (very low birth weight) babies is not replacing human milk
  - PKU (breastfeeding is still possible with phenylalanine-free formula supplementation and monitoring of PKU levels)

Potential for Contamination

- The product may be contaminated with aluminum or bacteria.
- Babies are at risk for contaminated water, mixing errors, and bacteria from ABM left at room temperature for too long.

Increased Health Risk to Babies

- ABM increases the risk of late neonatal hypocalcemia and dehydration.
- ABM can increase rates of allergy after a single feeding in the first days of life.
- Cow's milk protein is the most common food allergen in infants.
- Cow's milk allergy can occur as early as one week after introduction of ABM.
- ABM increases the incidence of atopic dermatitis and eczema in infants.
- Soy formula can change menstrual patterns and cause neurological deficits and renal problems.

Maternal Nutrition
Basic Nutrients

- Carbohydrates are the main source of energy for all body functions and activity.

  - **Simple carbohydrates** include sugar, jams, honey, chocolate, and other sweets.
  - **Complex carbohydrates** include starches such as cereals, rice, breads, crackers, pasta, vegetables, and fruits.

- Proteins are the major source of building material for internal organs, muscles, blood, skin, hair, and nails.

  - Proteins consist of 22 building blocks (amino acids). The diet must supply 8 essential amino acids.
  - **Complete protein foods** (most meats and dairy products) contain all the essential amino acids.
  - **Incomplete protein foods** (most vegetables or plants such as beans and grains) are lacking or extremely low in an essential amino acid.

- Fats are the most concentrated source of energy in the diet.

  - Fats are carriers for fat-soluble vitamins A, D, E, and K.
  - Prolonged digestion creates a longer lasting sensation of fullness.
  - Fatty acids give fats their different flavors, textures, and melting points.
  - **Saturated fatty acids** are derived from animal sources such as meat, milk products, and eggs.

- **Unsaturated fatty acids** are derived from vegetable, nut, and seed sources.
- A healthy diet should contain a greater amount of unsaturated fats than saturated fats.
- A diet low in fat is usually not appropriate during pregnancy and lactation.

- Vitamins convert fat and carbohydrates into energy and help to form bone and tissues.

  - The diet must provide necessary vitamins.
  - Excess amounts of some vitamins, such as vitamin A, can be harmful.
  - High doses of vitamin B_6 (600 mg/day) may cause lactation suppression.
  - Water-soluble vitamins (Bs and C) need to be replenished daily; maternal intake can affect the amount for most of these vitamins in her milk.
  - Folic acid contributes to cell growth and reproduction and can be obtained from leafy green vegetables and whole grains.
  - Fat-soluble vitamins (A, D, E, and K) are stored in the body's fatty tissues.

    - Vitamin A contributes to skeletal growth and maintains mucous membranes and keen sight.
    - Human milk is not deficient in vitamin D.

      - The human body is intended to make vitamin D through sunlight exposure.
      - Vitamin D deficiency is sunlight deficiency.

    - Vitamin K is essential for blood clotting; babies usually receive vitamin K by injection after birth.

- Minerals contribute to overall mental and physical well-being.

  - The diet must supply essential minerals.

    - Minerals help maintain physiological processes, strengthen skeletal structures, and preserve the vigor of the heart, the brain, and the muscle and nervous systems.
    - Minerals are important in hormone production.
    - Minerals help maintain water balance essential to mental and physical processes.

  - Calcium:

    - Calcium gives bones their rigidity and teeth their hardness.
    - Calcium has a role in blood clotting and controlling action of the heart, muscles, and nerves.
    - Pregnancy and lactation require high amounts of calcium (see Table 5-1 for sources of calcium).

- Iron:

  ‣ Pregnancy requires sufficient iron. Women who begin pregnancy with good iron stores and eat a varied diet do not need iron supplements.
  ‣ **Heme iron** comes from meat, poultry, and fish, and is easily absorbed.
  ‣ **Nonheme iron** comes from vegetables, iron-enriched cereals, and whole grains.
  ‣ Excess calcium can reduce iron absorption.

- Salt:

  ‣ Pregnancy requires more salt for the body to function well.
  ‣ Salt usually causes the body to retain fluid in the bloodstream.

Table 5-1 Good Sources of Calcium

Food	Calcium (mgs per serving)
Yogurt, plain (8 oz)	415
Cheddar cheese (2 oz)	408
Sardines, drained (3 oz)	372
American cheese (2 oz)	348
Yogurt, fruit-flavored (8 oz)	345
Milk, whole, low-fat, or skim (8 oz)	300
Watercress (1 cup chopped)	189
Chocolate pudding, instant (1/2 cup)	187
Collards (1/2 cup cooked)	179
Buttermilk pancakes (3–4 inches)	174
Pink salmon, canned (3 oz)	167
Tofu (4 oz)	145
Turnip greens (1/2 cup cooked)	134
Kale (1/2 cup cooked)	103
Shrimp, canned (3 oz)	99
Ice cream (1/2 cup)	88
Okra (1/2 cup cooked)	74
Rutabaga, mashed (1/2 cup cooked)	71
Broccoli (1/2 cup cooked)	68
Soybeans (1/2 cup cooked)	66
Cottage cheese (1/2 cup)	63
Bread, white or whole wheat (2 slices)	48

- Water:

  ◗ Water is the most abundant and important nutrient in the body.
  ◗ Pregnant and lactating women need to consume additional water.
  ◗ Thirst should dictate water consumption.
  ◗ Excessive water consumption can reduce milk production.

Nutrition Education

- Teach women about practical food choices rather than nutrients.
- Women are most receptive to nutrition education during pregnancy and lactation.

  - Sugary foods cause erratic blood sugar, fatigue, dizziness, nervousness, and headache.
  - Complex carbohydrates take longer to digest and prevent food cravings.
  - Fats create a longer feeling of fullness.
  - Food additives and processing alter nutritional quality favorably and unfavorably.
  - Vegetarian diets that include milk and eggs supply necessary nutrients.

- Nutrition in pregnancy:

  - A woman's body stores and the foods she eats provide energy and nutrients for her baby.
  - Pregnancy requires increased calcium, iron, and water intake.
  - Folic acid helps prevent anemia in pregnancy.
  - A newborn's vitamin K levels are low, and infants typically are supplemented.
  - Low levels of vitamin D in pregnancy result in low levels in the baby.

- Nutrition in lactation

  - A normal healthy diet will meet the mother's needs during lactation.
  - Protein is needed for hormone formation and milk production during lactation.
  - Lactation requires increased calcium, iron, and water intake.
  - Consuming excessive fluid can reduce milk production.
  - Lactation uses energy from body stores and from the mother's diet.
  - Well-nourished, healthy, lactating women can safely lose up to 1 pound per week.
  - Occasional alcohol timed around breastfeeding has not proven harmful to breastfed infants. Wait 2 to 3 hours after each drink or until effects of the alcohol are no longer felt.
  - Infants sensitive to caffeine may experience fussiness or excessive wakefulness.
  - Most foods are acceptable unless they cause allergic reactions in the mother or father or are consumed in excessive amounts.

SCIENCE OF LACTATION

ADVICE TO CLINICIANS
TEACH MOTHERS

- ▶ Strive for diet improvement of three well-balanced meals a day with snacks as needed.
- ▶ Eat small frequent meals, avoid fatty foods, drink plenty of liquids, and avoid highly spiced and very rich foods.
- ▶ Use the USDA food pyramid for meal planning.
- ▶ Balance complete protein and incomplete protein foods.
- ▶ Consume more unsaturated fats than saturated fats.
- ▶ Respond to thirst for necessary additional fluids.
- ▶ Protein and complex carbohydrates at breakfast will avoid later fatigue.
- ▶ Read food labels for nutritional information.
- ▶ A healthy diet helps overcome a fussy baby, recurring breast problems, infections or nipple soreness, depression, and lack of energy.

Tutorial for Students and Interns

Key Clinical Management Strategies

From *Clinical Guidelines for the Establishment of Exclusive Breastfeeding*, ILCA, 2005.

- Identify any maternal and infant contraindications to breastfeeding.
- Confirm that mothers understand the physiology of milk production, especially the role of milk removal.

Key Clinical Competencies

From *Clinical Competencies for IBCLC Practice* available at www.iblce.org.

- ☐ Perform a breast evaluation related to lactation.
- ☐ Instruct the mother about how milk is produced and the supply maintained, including discussion of growth and appetite spurts.
- ☐ Instruct the mother about assessment of adequate milk intake by the baby.
- ☐ Instruct the mother about normal infant sucking patterns.
- ☐ Instruct the mother about importance of exclusive breastmilk feeds and possible consequences of mixed feedings with cow milk or soy.
- ☐ Educate the mother about drugs (such as nicotine, alcohol, caffeine, and illicit drugs) and folk remedies (such as herbal teas).
- ☐ Assist mothers with medications compatible with breastfeeding.

☐ Assist mothers with lactose overload.
☐ Assist mothers with safe formula preparation and feeding techniques.

From Theory to Practice
Breast Anatomy

1. How would you respond to a pregnant woman who is concerned that her nipples are inverted and she may not be able to breastfeed? What anticipatory guidance can you give her for feedings?
2. What is the purpose of Montgomery glands?
3. Explain the correlation between suckling, nipple innervation, and skin layers.
4. How is the lymph system involved in engorgement?
5. Describe how the alveoli are involved in milk production and release.
6. How can you use your understanding of glandular development in the breast to explain why an adolescent woman is capable of full lactation?
7. How does a galactocele differ from an intraductal papilloma?
8. What signs would you look for in determining if a mother is at risk for insufficient milk production?
9. Which type(s) of breast surgery offer the greatest chance of successful lactation?

Breast Physiology

10. When does each stage of lactogenesis occur?
11. How is the breast fullness that accompanies stage II lactogenesis different from engorgement?
12. Explain the difference between the roles prolactin and oxytocin play in lactation.
13. How do breastfeeding patterns affect prolactin level?
14. What does "feedback inhibitor of lactation" mean, and how is it associated with breastfeeding patterns?
15. How does the prolactin inhibitor factor work?
16. What is the role of milk ejection relative to foremilk and hindmilk?
17. How would you approach a woman who is concerned that her milk is not letting down? What would be your first statement to her?
18. Which of the hormonal anomalies place mothers at risk for insufficient milk production?

Milk Transfer

19. What are the differences between nutritive and nonnutritive sucking?
20. Describe the typical sucking pattern from beginning to end of a feed.
21. How would you describe the process of milk transfer to an adolescent mother?

22. What does a mother need to understand about the relationship between her baby's suckling behavior and milk transfer?
23. What are the consequences of failing to drain the breast regularly, to both the mother and the baby?
24. How can you help a mother avoid the consequences of ineffective suckling for herself and her baby?
25. What breastfeeding practices will ensure that a baby receives adequate milk transfer?
26. A mother tells you she is concerned that her baby frequently sucks on his fist after feedings. She is worried that her baby is not receiving sufficient amounts of milk at feedings. What would you investigate? What would be your first statement to her?

Infant Nutrition

27. What is the importance of colostrum to a newborn?
28. What explains the difference in appearance between colostrum and mature milk?
29. Which protective properties in human milk are related to the infant's digestion?
30. Why is the mineral content of human milk more favorable to an infant than that of cow's milk?
31. What are the recommendations regarding vitamin D supplementation for a breastfeeding infant?
32. What are the differences between the milk of a woman who delivers prematurely and one who delivers at term?
33. A mother placed her expressed milk in the refrigerator 5 days ago and doesn't need to use it. She asks if she can freeze it and how long she can keep it frozen since she didn't put it in the freezer right after she expressed it. How do you respond? How would your response differ if her baby is in the NICU?
34. How would you respond to a mother who asks if there are any medications she cannot take?
35. What are the current guidelines for alcohol consumption by mothers who are breastfeeding?
36. Why is there so much conflicting information about impurities in human milk?
37. What role would supplemental feedings play in the effect a drug has on a breastfed infant?
38. How susceptible are infants to cow's milk protein allergy?
39. Under what circumstances would it be appropriate for a hypoglycemic infant to receive artificial formula?

Maternal Nutrition

40. What are the effects of maternal malnutrition during pregnancy and lactation?
41. What are a woman's special nutritional needs during lactation? How would you help a mother with a nutrition plan to ensure she meets her needs?
42. How would you advise a woman who wishes to lose weight while she is lactating? What practical suggestions can you offer to her?
43. What information can you use to motivate a woman to improve her diet?
44. How would you approach a mother who is a chronic smoker and plans to smoke during lactation?
45. What precautions would you share with a mother who is a vegetarian? What do you need to learn from her in order to provide appropriate suggestions?
46. How can a woman achieve optimal nutrition on a restricted income?
47. How can maternal consumption of caffeine affect a breastfed infant?

CHAPTER 6

Assessment

In This Chapter

Newborn Assessment

Posture

- Healthy tone:

  - Arms and legs are in moderate flexion.
  - The baby resists having his extremities extended.
  - The fists are closed and usually near the face.
  - Held in the ventral position, the baby alternates between trying to raise and lower his head.

- Hypotonia—very low body tone:

  - Extremities are in extension with little resistance to passive movement.

    - The baby appears floppy, sluggish, and flaccid.
    - Held in the ventral position, the baby droops and is unable to raise his head.
    - The baby may have difficulty staying latched onto the breast due to a weak suck.
    - The baby frequently nurses with his shoulders elevated to just beneath his ears in an effort to support his neck and chin.

  - A baby who is premature or who has Down syndrome will show some degree of hypotonia.

- Hypertonia—very rigid body tone:

    - The baby is often in hyperextension, arching away from the breast and the mother.
    - The baby pulls away from contact and does not snuggle into the mother's chest or neck.
    - The baby is often very alert and squirmy and holds his head erect from a prone position or on the shoulder.
    - Held in the ventral position, the baby is straight and lifts his head and buttocks on a horizontal plane.
    - A baby with neurological damage may be hypertonic.

Skin

- Healthy newborn skin is warm and dry.

    - It has a pink or ruddy appearance from increased red blood cells.
    - There are minimal subcutaneous fat deposits.
    - It springs back when grasped between a finger and thumb and released.

- Normal variations occur in skin tone and appearance.

    - **Acrocyanosis** is a bluish tinge of the hands and feet.

        - It is caused by poor peripheral circulation, especially with exposure to cold.
        - Symptoms should disappear after a few days.

    - **Erythema toxicum** is a normal newborn rash that is a pink to red macular (raised) area with a yellow or white center.

        - It is common on a newborn's trunk or limbs.
        - It appears 1 to 2 days after birth and usually disappears within 1 week.
        - There is no apparent significance or need for treatment.

    - **Infant acne** appears on the face, primarily on the nose, forehead, and cheeks.

        - It is a normal response to maternal hormones.
        - It starts at about 2 weeks of age and disappears at 8 to 10 weeks.

    - **Diaper rash** is a reddened, small, pimplelike rash.

        - A shiny, red, flat rash that does not respond may result from a yeast infection.
        - Skin that is chafed or has pustules may result from a bacterial infection.
        - Wash the buttocks and apply zinc oxide.

- **Dehydration** is characterized by loose skin that slowly returns to its original position.

  ‣ Yellowing in skin color is caused by increased bilirubin.
  ‣ Dry, flaky, or peeling skin is normal and is not a sign of dehydration.

Head, Neck, and Shoulders

- **Molding** is an overriding of the newborn's skull bones.

  - The baby's head may appear asymmetric.
  - Severe molding can cause temporary latching difficulty.

- **Caput succedaneum** is swelling caused by a collection of fluid between the skin and cranial bone.

  - Swelling begins to subside soon after birth.
  - The area is sensitive to touch.

- A **cephalhematoma** is swelling from pooled blood between the head and periosteum.

  - Swelling slowly becomes larger in the first few days after birth. It does not cross the sagittal suture lines.
  - Bilirubin levels may increase.
  - It takes about 6 weeks to resolve completely and is sensitive to touch.

- The **fontanel** is the space between the bones of the skull covered by tough membranes.

  - The anterior fontanel remains soft until about 18 months.
  - The posterior fontanel closes at about 2 months.
  - A soft, sunken fontanel is a sign of dehydration.

- Facial asymmetry may result from injury to nerves due to birth trauma.

  - The baby's tongue may be off center in his mouth.
  - Position the nipple over the center of the baby's tongue rather than the mouth.
  - Asymmetry will resolve over several days following birth.

- Eyes

  - Swelling of the eyelids recedes in a few days.
  - Scleral hemorrhages may be seen.
  - Jaundice in the white portion of the eye indicates a bilirubin level above 5.
  - Final eye color is established by 6 to 12 months of age.

- Neck

    - The newborn's neck is very short and too weak to provide head support.
    - **Torticollis** is a shortening of the muscle from the base of the ear to the clavicle.

        ‣ The baby keeps his head twisted to the side, usually to the right.
        ‣ Breastfeeding may only be comfortable with the head turned to the side.
        ‣ The football hold provides control over neck position.
        ‣ The side lying position provides postural support.
        ‣ The baby may need referral for physical therapy.

- Clavicle fracture is a common birth trauma.

    - It may restrict the use of the baby's arm.
    - The baby may resist breastfeeding in a position that places pressure on the fractured area.
    - The fracture heals quickly within about 3 weeks.

Oral Cavity

- The baby's oral cavity is extremely sensitive.

    - Visual inspection is preferred over digital.
    - Gum lines should be smooth.
    - The palate should be intact and gently arched.
    - The tongue should be able to extend over the lower alveolar ridge and up to the middle of the baby's mouth.

- The **sublingual frenulum** is the fold of skin under the tongue that controls motion. A short frenulum (**ankyloglossia**) can prevent adequate extension of the tongue.

    - The tip of the tongue has a heart-shaped appearance when extended.
    - Chronic nipple soreness, slow weight gain, low milk supply, mastitis, or plugged ducts can occur.
    - Clipping the frenulum will enable the baby to extend the tongue adequately.

- The **labial frenum** is the fold of skin that anchors the upper lip to the top gum. A prominent frenum results in a gap between the two top front teeth.

    - The baby may have difficulty flanging the upper lip.
    - It may cause compression and discomfort or difficulty with latch.

- **Buccal pads**, fatty tissue in the cheeks, help decrease space within the mouth to increase negative pressure and facilitate milk transfer.

- They are not present in a malnourished or preterm infant.
- The mother can place her finger against the baby's cheeks to compensate for lack of fat pads (Dancer hand position).

- The **hard palate** is in the front of the mouth, and the *soft palate* lies behind it in line with the end of the upper alveolar ridge.

  - **High, arched, or bubble palate:**

    - The nipple may "catch" in the groove and not elongate.
    - It is difficult for the tongue to compress the lactiferous ducts adequately.
    - Nipple soreness, long feedings, poor weight gain, and an unsatisfied infant can result.

  - **Cleft palate:**

    - The baby may choke and gag while nursing.
    - Milk may escape from the baby's nose when milk flow is strong.
    - Feeding in an upright position at the breast often helps.
    - In a **submucosal cleft**, skin covers a cleft of the hard or soft palate.
    - Feedings will be long and additional pumping may be necessary to maintain an adequate milk supply.

- **Thrush** (candidiasis) most frequently occurs because of *Candida albicans*.

  - White patches appear between the baby's gums and lips, on the inside of the cheeks, or on the tongue.
  - The patches cannot be removed without causing bleeding.
  - It transfers to the mother's nipples, and the mother and baby must be treated simultaneously.
  - Thrush can be present without visible signs.

Reflexes

- The **Moro (startle) reflex** encourages gentle handling of baby.
- The **grasp reflex** assists the baby in crawling to the breast.
- **Arching** helps the baby pull away if his face is pushed into the breast.
- **Bauer's response** is spontaneous crawling motion and head extension when pressure is exerted on the soles of the baby's feet.
- **Rooting** causes the baby to turn his head in the direction of a stimulus to the cheek. The baby's mouth opens and the tongue comes forward.
- **Sucking** is elicited when the nipple reaches the juncture between the hard and soft palates.

ASSESSMENT

Digestion
Burping

- Burping helps bring air bubbles in the milk to the top of the baby's stomach to be expelled.
- Burping decreases gas pains and reduces the possibility of spitting up.
- Burp a crying baby before putting him to breast.
- Feeding before the baby is ravenous reduces the amount of air the baby takes in.
- Holding the baby at a 45° angle after feedings will help bring up air.

Spitting Up

- Babies can spit up often during the early months.

  - There may be mucus in the baby's stomach.
  - Too much time lapses between feedings and the baby is overanxious and gulps air.
  - The baby is overfeeding or milk production is overactive.

- **Projectile vomiting** is a violent expulsion of milk that travels several feet and may be a sign of pyloric stenosis.

  - **Pyloric stenosis** may begin suddenly when the baby is several weeks old.
  - Vomiting may get progressively worse with a decreasing number of wet diapers.
  - The outflow valve of the baby's stomach does not open adequately.
  - It may indicate an obstruction of the intestines or a strangulated hernia.
  - Pyloric stenosis requires careful medical observation and possible surgery.

Gastroesophageal Reflux Disease (GERD)

- GERD may cause the baby to spit up and can lead to poor weight gain.
- GERD causes burning and discomfort; human milk is not as irritating as formula.
- Medication can decrease stomach acid and help milk pass more quickly into the intestines.
- Cow's milk allergy from the mother's diet or supplemental formula may be a cause.
- GERD usually subsides by 1 year of age.
- Feed frequently and from only one breast at a feeding.

  - This limits the amount of milk the baby takes in at a feeding.
  - The baby feeds long enough to receive the fatty hindmilk at the end of the feed.
  - The baby is able to digest and retain more of the milk.

- Feed with the baby in an upright position so gravity helps the milk stay down.
- Hold the baby upright after feeding.

Output

- Voiding frequency in the first week of life should increase daily.

  - Urine should be pale yellow to clear in color.
  - Pink (copper or brick dust) stains are not significant in the first 1 to 3 days; assess hydration status if it occurs later than 3 days.
  - By 4 to 5 days, the baby should void at least 6 times in 24 hours.

- Stooling begins with black, tarry **meconium**, which passes within the first 24 to 36 hours.

  - Color transitions to greenish black, to greenish brown, to brown, and then to golden or mustard yellow color by 48 to 72 hours.
  - Texture of stools ranges from watery, to seedy yellow, to toothpaste consistency.
  - The baby should stool at least 3 or more times in 24 hours in the first month.

    - By 4 to 6 weeks of age, frequency will decrease.
    - Older babies may range from several stools daily or once every 3 days.
    - Infrequent stooling in the first month of life needs to be explored.

      - It is usually due to insufficient intake of milk or the baby not receiving hindmilk.
      - Nursing more frequently resolves most infrequent stooling problems.
      - Weigh, examine, and monitor the baby for adequate intake.

    - **Hirschsprung's disease** may cause infrequent stooling; monitor the baby carefully.

      - An exclusively breastfed infant gains weight but does not stool frequently.
      - Part of the baby's intestines lacks proper innervation and the stool cannot pass easily.
      - The baby may have a large, bloated abdomen from a collection of stool and gas.

  - Constipation produces stools that are molded and firm to the touch.

    - Constipation is rare in breastfed infants.
    - Discontinuing iron supplements for a few days allows the baby's system to return to normal.
    - If the baby is old enough to receive them, yogurt, oatmeal, or prune juice may help.

- Diarrhea produces stools that are watery, greenish, or foul smelling. It may indicate illness or a reaction to antibiotics taken by the mother or baby.

Behavior
Approach and Avoidance Behaviors

- Approach behaviors invite interaction with the baby.

  - Extending his tongue
  - Placing his hands on his face
  - Sounds such as a whimper
  - Clasping his hands or feet
  - Folding his fingers
  - Moving his body, including curling or turning his trunk or shoulders
  - Bringing his hand to his mouth
  - Grasping movements
  - Extending his legs or feet
  - Mouthing movements
  - Opening his mouth and making sucking movements
  - Holding the caregiver's hand
  - Pursing his lips
  - Locking visually or auditorily

- Withdrawal or avoidance behaviors discourage interaction with the baby.

  - Spitting up
  - Gagging or hiccoughing
  - Grunting or straining
  - Grimacing or retracting his lip
  - Arching his trunk away
  - Splaying his fingers
  - Extending his arms like an airplane
  - Extending his arms or legs into midair
  - Sneezing, yawning, sighing, or coughing
  - Averting his eyes
  - Frowning
  - Startling

Feeding Behaviors and Readiness

- A baby progresses through a series of feeding behaviors.

  - He begins to wriggle and his closed eyes exhibit rapid eye movement.
  - He passes one or both hands over his head and brings his hand to his mouth.

- He makes sucking motions, and if his cheek or mouth is touched, he begins to root.
- More vigorous sucking begins.
- He settles back into a less active state.
- He cries if signals are unheeded or falls back asleep without feeding.

- Interest in feeding depends on the baby's level of alertness.

  - Most babies move from deep to light sleep in 20 to 30 minutes.
  - Feeding behavior may be evident during the light sleep, drowsy, and quiet alert states.
  - The baby may exhibit feeding behavior several times in a span of 20 to 30 minutes.

Disposition

- An **average baby** is quiet, alert, and listening when awake.

  - He nurses 8–12 times in 24 hours.
  - He sleeps 12–20 hours a day with one or two longer periods balanced by one or two fussy periods.
  - He is responsive when handled and learns self-soothing.

- An **easy baby** is less demanding with relatively no fussiness.

  - He nurses 8–12 times in 24 hours.
  - He sleeps for longer periods.
  - He needs tactile stimulation and attention for emotional and physical development.

- A **placid baby** is quietly alert and tranquil when awake, making few demands for attention.

  - He may request as few as 4–6 feedings in 24 hours.
  - He may not demonstrate feeding behavior and falls back asleep.

    - A noise device will alert the mother when the baby awakes and moves about.
    - The mother can set an alarm to check the baby every 2–3 hours and pick him up when awake.

  - He typically gains weight slowly and needs monitoring for undernourishment.
  - He sleeps 18–20 hours a day.
  - He may become withdrawn and lethargic and needs tactile stimulation and attention for emotional and physical development.
  - Avoid pacifying techniques. The mother needs to be aggressive in feeding attempts.

- An **active and fussy** baby is active and unable to self-soothe when awake.

  - He may nurse more frequently because of a greater need for comfort.
  - May seem insatiable at the breast and impatient for the milk to let down.
  - He will sleep fewer hours and may have several periods of inconsolable crying.
  - He may overreact to freedom and stimulation.

    - Use gentle, slow movements.
    - Keep him warm and swaddled to avoid startling.
    - Hold him often and close to the mother's body.

  - He may respond well to nursing, dozing, and playing at the breast for generous periods.
  - He may spit up often from being overly full.

    - Limit him to one breast at a feeding so he can nurse on a drained breast for comfort.
    - He may need to be burped often.

Fussiness

- Crying

  - Babies cry from hunger when feeding behavior is unheeded.

    - Crying is often more prevalent in the evening when cluster feeding is common.
    - A newborn cries from hunger usually 1½ to 2 hours or more after a feeding.
    - To determine if crying is from hunger, consider:

      - How long it has been since the last feeding and how long the baby fed
      - The baby's general disposition and ability to be soothed
      - Feeding behavior the baby demonstrated

  - Babies cry from discomfort for several reasons.

    - A wet or soiled diaper cools against the baby's skin.
    - The baby is too warm; dress him in the same type of clothing that an adult would wear.
    - Being undressed causes a loss of a warm secure feeling.
    - The texture of clothing or a blanket causes irritation.
    - The baby has a heat rash or diaper rash.
    - The baby is uncomfortable from gas or being overly full.
    - The baby reacts to sudden movement, touch, smell, light, noise, or excessive handling.

Comfort measures for crying:

▶ Constant, soft, soothing noise
▶ Swaddling and being held
▶ Wearing the baby in a sling
▶ Recreating the sounds and feeling of the womb
▶ Firm touch and gentle stroking
▶ Massage the baby's stomach, shoulders, head, hands, feet, and back. Then hold the baby against the shoulder and soothe him until he calms.

- Coliclike behavior:

  - Spasmodic contractions of smooth muscle cause pain and discomfort.
  - A rumbling sound may be audible in the baby's gut.
  - Symptoms generally subside by 16 weeks of age.
  - The baby exhibits unexplained fussiness, fretfulness, and irritability.
  - The baby expresses severe discomfort most of the time.
  - The baby's cries are piercing and explosive attacks.
  - The baby may draw up his legs sharply, clench his fists, appear intense, and be easily startled.
  - The baby may grimace, stiffen, twist his body, and awaken easily and frequently.

- Possible causes of colic symptoms:

  - The mother and child feel stress and tension.
  - The baby has allergies.
  - The mother has hyperemesis, pelvic pain, or distress during pregnancy.
  - The baby has an immature gastrointestinal and/or neurological system.

    ▸ Peristalsis is irregular, faint, forceful, or spasmodic.
    ▸ Lack of muscle tone allows food to move from the stomach down into the intestines.
    ▸ The colon contracts violently during feedings.

  - The mother's progesterone level drops 1 to 2 weeks after birth.
  - The milk contains high levels of motilin, a digestive hormone that stimulates muscle contractions.
  - There were intrauterine or birth-related problems such as prematurity, small for gestational age, birth trauma, or anoxia.
  - The mother had hypertension, epidural anesthesia, distress during pregnancy, or a birth intervention.

Signs of food sensitivity:

▶ Frequently pulling off the breast and arching and crying while feeding

▶ Stuffy or drippy nose without signs of a cold

▶ Itchy nose

▶ Red, scaly, oily rash on the forehead or eyebrows, in the hair, or behind the ears

▶ Eczema

▶ Red rectal ring

▶ Fretful sleeping or persistent sleeplessness

▶ Frequent spitting up or vomiting

▶ Diarrhea or green stools, perhaps with blood in them

▶ Wheezing

- The mother used heroin, marijuana, barbiturates, or cocaine prenatally.
- One of the parents smokes.
- The baby suffers from lactose overload because of an overactive letdown, over-abundant milk production, or insufficient hindmilk intake.
- The baby has food sensitivity.

Sleep

- Sleep periods range from 8 to 20 hours per day.

  - Variations are developmental, environmental, or nutritional.
  - Excessive tiredness or stimulation can cause fretfulness before and during sleep.
  - Sounds, lights, temperature of the room and bedding, and low humidity can interfere with sleep.
  - Babies who sleep separated from their mothers may wake more at night.
- A baby may have trouble sleeping if the mother consumes too much caffeine.

Sources of food sensitivity:

▶ Cow and soy milk intolerance (eliminate dairy foods for 2 weeks and gradually reintroduce slowly)

▶ Infant vitamins, fluoride, iron supplements, or antibiotics that inflame the intestinal lining (leaky gut syndrome)

▶ Maternal medications, vitamin supplements, caffeine, high-protein foods, milk, wheat, chocolate, eggs, or nuts

- Parents can encourage their baby to sleep.

    - Establish a bedtime ritual with quiet, soothing activities and nursing.
    - Warm the sleeping area before putting the baby in bed.
    - Use flannel sheets on the baby's bed.
    - Place a night light in the room to avoid turning on a light when the baby wakes at night.
    - Change the baby's diaper before nursing on the second breast.
    - Wake the baby to nurse every 2–3 hours during the day.

- Mothers can enhance their sleep.

    - Sleep when the baby sleeps.
    - Go to bed early and take the baby to bed with her.
    - Ask her partner to bring the baby to the bed for nursing during the night.

- Parents can create a safe sleep environment (see Figure 6-1).

    - Place the newborn in a supine position and in close proximity to the parents for sleep.
    - Safe cobedding has health advantages.

        ▸ The mother's warmth and familiar smell comfort the baby and allow access for feeding.
        ▸ Babies arouse more often and in synchrony with their mothers, reducing the risk of SIDS and promoting nighttime nursing.
        ▸ Mothers and babies receive more total sleep.
        ▸ Most mothers instinctively recognize their babies' presence and respond.

Growth

- Assess overall pattern of weight gain, gain since the previous weight check, and the lowest weight.

    - Record the baby's growth in length and in an increase in head circumference.
    - Monitor alertness, skin turgor, moist mucous membranes, and adequate output.
    - See Appendix G for the World Health Organization growth charts for breastfed babies.

- Babies regulate their food intake when there are no arbitrary limits on feeding.

    - Giving water to breastfed babies can affect their caloric intake.
    - Energy needs correspond to age and activity.

Creating a Safe Infant Sleep Environment

Adapted from Infant Sleep Environment Safety Checklist by Patricia Donohue-Carey, BS, LCCE, CLE. Solitary or Shared Sleep: What's Safe? *Mothering*; 44–47 September/October 2002. Printed with permission.

Precautions for crib and adult beds:
- Use a firm mattress to avoid suffocation.
- Have no gaps between the mattress and the frame.
- Keep bedding tight around the mattress.
- Avoid strings or ties on the baby's and parents' night clothes.
- Avoid soft items such as comforters, pillows, featherbeds, stuffed animals, lambskins, and bean bags.
- Keep the baby's face uncovered to allow ventilation.
- Put the baby on his back to sleep.
- Do not overheat the room or overdress the baby.
- Do not place a crib near window cords or sashes.

Additional precautions for cribs:
- When the baby learns to sit, lower the mattress level to avoid falling or climbing out.
- When the baby learns to stand, set the mattress level at its lowest point and remove crib bumpers.
- When the baby reaches a height of 35 inches or the side rail is less than three quarters of his height, move the baby to another bed.
- Crib bumpers should have at least six ties, no longer than 6 inches.
- Hang crib mobiles well out of reach and remove when the baby can sit or reach.
- Remove crib gyms when the baby can get up on all fours.

Additional precautions for cosleeping:
- Parents pull back and fasten long hair.
- Do not use alcohol or other drugs, including over-the-counter or prescription medications.
- Have no head/foot board railings with spaces wider than allowed in safety-approved cribs.
- Use no bed rails with infants less than one year.
- Do not allow siblings in bed with a the baby less than 1 year old.
- Do not cosleep in a waterbed.
- Avoid placing the bed directly alongside furniture or a wall.

Additional precautions regarding infant sleep:
- Do not sleep with the baby on sofas or overstuffed chairs.
- Do not put the baby to sleep alone in an adult bed.
- Do not place the baby to sleep in car or infant seats.

Figure 6-1 Creating a Safe Infant Sleep Environment.

Sources: American Academy of Pediatrics policy statement, *Changing Concepts of Sudden Infant Death Syndrome: Implications for Infant Sleeping Environments and Sleep Position* (RE9956); March 2000. Available at: www.aap.org/policyRe9946.html.

American Academy of Pediatrics. *Caring for Your Baby and Young Child, Birth to Age 5* (New York: Bantam Books, 1998), 16–17.

SIDS Alliance. *Safe Infant Bedding Practices.* Available at: www.sidsalliance.org/Healthcare/default.asp.

- ▸ Energy needs at birth are 115 kcal/kg/day.
- ▸ Energy needs at 6 months are 82 kcal/kg/day.
- ▸ Caloric needs rise slightly as the baby becomes active and mobile.

- Loss of fluids and passage of meconium cause the newborn to lose up to 7% of birth weight.

  - Excessive intravenous fluids for the mother may artificially increase the baby's birth weight and result in large voids and weight loss in the first 24 hours.
  - A weight loss of more than 7% requires evaluation and possible assistance (see Appendix H).
  - By day 3, a full term infant should not lose any more weight.
  - By the end of the first week, weight loss should stabilize.
  - By 10–14 days, the baby should have regained birth weight.

- A baby gains weight more rapidly in the first 2–3 months and weighs less from 6–12 months than a formula-fed baby weighs.

Breast Assessment
Examining a Mother's Breasts

- Ensure privacy, ask permission, and obtain a signed consent if required.
- Be aware of cultural customs of modesty.
- Ask about changes in breast size and areola darkening in both breasts during pregnancy to determine sufficient functioning tissue.
- Examine both breasts at the same time to observe symmetry.
- Note the skin's elasticity, engorgement, lumps, swelling, or redness.
- Look for evidence of past breast surgery that may have severed ducts or nerves.
- Note the size and shape of the nipples and the size and graspability of the areola.
- Learn how nipples respond to cold or touch to determine their ability to evert.

Lumps in the Breast

- The normal lactating breast is lumpy due to enlarged milk-filled alveoli.

  - Other lumps may be due to a plugged duct or breast infection.
  - Fibrocystic lumps shrink and become less noticeable after menstruation.

- A **galactocele** is a cyst caused by the closing or blockage of a milk duct.

  - It contains a thick, creamy milklike substance that may ooze when compressed.

ASSESSMENT

- It can be aspirated or removed surgically to prevent refilling; breastfeeding may continue.

- An **intraductal papilloma** is a benign, nontender tumor within a milk duct.

  - It is usually associated with a spontaneous bloody discharge from one breast.
  - It can be removed surgically; breastfeeding may continue.

- A lump that does not move downward and break up may be a result of malignancy.

  - A baby may refuse to nurse from a cancerous breast.
  - Breastfeeding can continue after a biopsy.

    - Milk may leak from a biopsy incision site
    - Healing may require temporary interruption of breastfeeding.

  - Breastfeeding may not be compatible with treatment for breast cancer.
  - **Paget's disease** is a malignancy of the breast that is usually unilateral.

    - It produces a scaly, itchy skin condition on the nipple and areola that mimics eczema.
    - There may be a bloody discharge from the nipple and a lump in the breast.
    - The nipple may appear flattened.

Breastfeeding Assessment

Note: See Chapter 9 for problem solving with latch or suckling difficulties.

Assessing Latch

- Principles of a good latch:

  - The baby is in a receptive state to settle and organize.
  - The baby turns his head toward the breast and opens his mouth wide.
  - The breast is slightly above center of the baby's open mouth.
  - The lips are flanged out and open wide at about a 140° angle.
  - The bottom lip covers most of the areola and the top lip covers somewhat less of the areola.
  - The latch is asymmetrical to ensure adequate compression of ducts.
  - The tongue is under the breast and extends over the alveolar ridge.
  - The baby takes in a large mouthful of breast tissue.
  - The tongue forms a trough for milk to flow.
  - The baby draws the nipple into the center of his mouth or tongue.

- The jaws are well behind the nipple and compress the milk ducts rhythmically.
- The baby maintains a hold on the breast and establishes a suck–swallow–breathe pattern.
- The mother feels no pain.

- Signs of a poor latch:

  - The baby is unable to stay on the breast for more than several sucks.
  - The mother has pain during or after feedings.
  - The baby's cheeks appear dimpled or puckered.
  - The breast slides in and out of the baby's mouth throughout sucking.
  - Clicking or smacking noises are heard when the baby suckles.
  - Little or no swallowing is evident during a feeding.
  - The baby is fussy during or after feedings.
  - The nipple appears flattened, creased, or blanched after the baby unlatches.
  - Little or no breast changes occur from the beginning to the end of a feeding after stage II lactogenesis.
  - The baby has inadequate voiding and/or stooling.

- Possible causes of latch difficulties:

  - It is common to have some difficulty in the first few days until the milk comes in.
  - The mother has breast or nipple abnormalities.
  - The mother has low back pain or carpal tunnel syndrome.
  - A perineal or cesarean incision from delivery causes pain.
  - The baby has a cleft lip or palate, neurological or orthopedic problem, Down syndrome, a fractured clavicle, ankyloglossia (tight frenulum), or a high palate.
  - The mother has a strong milk ejection reflex.
  - The mother has very large breasts.
  - The baby is late preterm (37–38 weeks) or small for gestational age.

- Consequences of a poor latch:

  - Incorrect latch is the primary cause of nipple soreness.
  - Anticipation of pain inhibits the milk ejection reflex.
  - The mother is at risk for engorgement, plugged ducts, and mastitis.
  - Milk production will diminish and lactation failure is likely.
  - The baby receives primarily foremilk resulting in increased hunger and fussiness.
  - Urine and stool output is inadequate.
  - The baby develops jaundice.
  - The baby fails to gain adequate weight or may even lose weight.
  - A need for supplements leads to early weaning.

Assessing Suckling

- Efficient milk transfer requires appropriate suckling.

  - Feeding begins with nonnutritive sucking, short jaw excursions, and brief sucks of two sucks per second to promote milk flow.
  - The pattern changes to nutritive sucking when milk is available, with wide jaw excursions and long, deep sucks of one suck per second.
  - The baby's gums alternately compress and release as milk flows.
  - The baby establishes a regular pattern of suck–swallow–breathe, alternating between nutritive and nonnutritive sucking throughout the feeding.

- A baby may have a weak or ineffective suck in the first few days of life.

  - Suckling usually improves with patience, practice, and proper positioning.
  - A baby who is sleepy or weak from insufficient nourishment may not suckle nutritively.
  - Most uncoordinated suckling resolves by increasing the baby's caloric intake.
  - Intubation or other birth interventions can delay development of a normal nutritive suck.
  - Ineffective suckling may result from sucking habits in utero or artificial nipple feedings.
  - A baby who is not suckling effectively needs to be supplemented until the issue is resolved.

Assessing Milk Transfer

- Signs of sufficient milk transfer:

  - The baby moves from short rapid sucks to slow deep sucks.
  - The mother notices signs of the milk ejection reflex.
  - Swallowing is evident after every one to four sucks.
  - The baby is able to maintain his latch throughout the feeding.
  - The breast softens as the feeding progresses (after stage II lactogenesis).
  - The baby spontaneously unlatches and is satiated.
  - The nipple is not blanched or compressed when the baby unlatches.

- Signs of sufficient milk intake:

  - The baby has six or more wet diapers per day by day 4.
  - The baby has three or more stools per day by day 4.
  - The baby is content between most feedings.
  - The baby has regular intervals of wakefulness, sleep, and feeding.
  - The baby has a healthy skin tone and color.
  - The baby has periods of alertness, engaging, and eye contact.

- Fat creases are evident in the baby's arms and legs, and the baby fills out his clothing.
- The baby has increases in length and head size and regular weight gain.

Tutorial for Students and Interns

Key Clinical Management Strategies

From *Clinical Guidelines for the Establishment of Exclusive Breastfeeding*, ILCA, 2005.

- Avoid using pacifiers, artificial nipples, and supplements, unless medically indicated.
- Identify maternal and infant risk factors that may affect the mother's or infant's ability to breastfeed effectively and provide appropriate assistance and follow-up.
- Assess the mother and infant for signs of effective breastfeeding and intervene if breastfeeding is ineffective.
- Assist the mother and infant in achieving a comfortable position and effective latch (attachment).
- Confirm that mothers understand normal breastfed infant behaviors and have realistic expectations regarding infant care and breastfeeding.
- Observe and document at least one breastfeeding in each 8-hour period during the postpartum period.
- Teach mothers to recognize and respond to early infant feeding cues and confirm that the baby feeds at least eight times in each 24 hours.
- If medically indicated, provide additional nutrition using a method of supplementation that is least likely to compromise transition to exclusive breastfeeding.

Key Clinical Competencies

From *Clinical Competencies for IBCLC Practice* available at www.iblce.org.

- ☐ Perform a comprehensive breastfeeding assessment.
- ☐ Perform a breast evaluation related to lactation.
- ☐ Assess and evaluate the infant's ability to breastfeed.
- ☐ Assess effective milk transfer.
- ☐ Assess contributing factors and etiology of problems.
- ☐ Identify correct latch (attachment).
- ☐ Identify the mother's concerns or problems, planned interventions, evaluation of outcomes and follow-up.
- ☐ Develop a breastfeeding risk assessment.
- ☐ Observe a feeding.

ASSESSMENT

☐ Instruct the mother about normal newborn behavior, including why, when and how to wake a sleepy newborn.

☐ Instruct the mother about normal infant sucking patterns.

☐ Instruct the mother about how milk is produced and supply maintained, including discussion of growth and appetite spurts.

☐ Instruct the mother about assessment of adequate milk intake by the baby.

☐ Assist mothers with care of their breasts.

☐ Instruct the mother about prevention and treatment of sore nipples.

☐ Instruct the mother about SIDS prevention behaviors.

☐ Assist mothers with breast surgery or trauma.

☐ Assist mothers with overproduction of milk.

☐ Assist mothers with ankyloglossia (short frenulum).

☐ Assist mothers with colic or fussiness.

☐ Assist mothers with gastric reflux.

☐ Calculate an infant's caloric and volume requirements.

☐ Demonstrate appropriate use and understanding of potential disadvantages or risks of use of a device to evert nipples.

From Theory to Practice
Newborn Assessment

1. What elements would you include in a feeding plan for a mother whose baby is hypotonic?

2. What elements would you include in a feeding plan for a mother whose baby is hypertonic?

3. What aspects of infant assessment would alert you to the possibility of dehydration?

4. How does assessment of the infant's head and face alert you to the potential for breastfeeding difficulties?

5. What aspects of the infant's oral anatomy can you assess through visual inspection alone?

6. What circumstances would indicate the need for digital inspection of the infant's oral cavity?

7. What are the potential consequences of a short frenulum or frenum for the mother? What are the potential consequences for the infant?

8. What role do the infant's buccal pads have in effective breastfeeding? What can a mother do to compensate for undeveloped buccal pads?

9. Why can a high, arched or bubble palate be problematic with breastfeeding?

10. What elements would you include in a feeding plan for a mother whose baby has a cleft palate?

11. Why is it important to treat both the mother and baby when only one has signs of a thrush infection?

12. Which infant reflexes are factors in effective breastfeeding and how are they involved?

13. When does spitting up indicate a need to make changes in breastfeeding management?
14. What feeding plan would you develop for an infant with gastroesophageal reflex?
15. What recommendations would you give to a mother for monitoring her baby's output?
16. How would you respond to a mother who is concerned that her 1-month-old baby has not had a bowel movement for the past 3 days?
17. What precautions would you give to parents about watching for feeding behavior?
18. What tips would you give to the mother of a placid baby regarding breast-feeding?
19. What tips would you give to the mother of a fussy baby regarding breast-feeding?
20. A mother tells you her 5-day-old infant has a lot of gas and cries after feedings. What would you investigate? What would be your first statement to her?
21. What feeding plan would you develop for the mother of a colicky baby?
22. How would you respond to a mother who wants to start giving her 4-month-old baby a bottle of formula in the evening so he will start sleeping longer at night?

Breast Assessment

23. What might you observe when assessing a mother's breasts that would alert you to potential problems with milk production?
24. How can you help a woman minimize the possibility that her inverted nipples will prevent her baby from obtaining a good latch for feeds?
25. What characteristics of a lump in the breast would alert you to the potential of a cancerous growth?

Breastfeeding Assessment

26. What aspects of a good latch make it less likely that an inverted nipple would present a problem with latch?
27. In what way does an asymmetrical latch improve breastfeeding?
28. Why do a baby's cheeks dimple or pucker with a poor latch?
29. Why does clicking or smacking indicate a poor latch?
30. How does a poor latch cause the nipple to slide in and out of the baby's mouth?
31. What aspect of a poor latch causes the nipple to appear flattened or creased after the baby unlatches? How does this affect milk transfer?
32. How does nonnutritive sucking differ from nutritive sucking?
33. What hospital interventions can interfere with a newborn's sucking effectiveness?
34. What sucking pattern would the mother of a 3-week-old baby want to observe during a feed?

35. What signs can a mother watch for during a feed that will indicate her baby is receiving adequate milk?
36. If you could tell a mother only three signs of sufficient milk intake, what would be the three most important signs to tell her?

CHAPTER 7

Facilitating Breastfeeding

In This Chapter

Birth and Postpartum Care

Labor and Delivery

- Limit the use of medications, anesthesia, and other birth interventions.

  - Epidural medications diminish early suckling and increase intrapartum fever.
  - Pitocin and IVs may cause breast and nipple edema and delay milk production.
  - Forceps and vacuum extraction increase the risk of bruising and pain.
  - Putting a baby to breast immediately after deep suctioning may cause breast aversion.

- Kangaroo care is more effective than a radiant warmer in maintaining temperature.
- Enable mothers to nurse directly after birth and offer help.

  - Bonding is strongest in the first 1 or 2 hours and is enhanced with skin-to-skin contact.
  - Rooting and sucking reflexes are particularly strong in the first 1 or 2 hours.
  - Delaying the first breastfeeding increases the use of artificial baby milk.

Physical Recovery Following Birth

- Discomfort:

    - The mother's abdomen still protrudes because of stretched muscles.
    - Walking may be more of a waddle because of loosened pelvic ligaments and stitches or pads.
    - Backaches may result from hormones having softened or loosened the sacroiliac ligaments.
    - The perineum is swollen and tender after a vaginal delivery.
    - Initial breast fullness may be slightly uncomfortable.
    - Incisional pain may cause discomfort in positioning.

- Body functions:

    - Energy level may be low.
    - The uterus decreases to about 1 pound by 1 week and to about 2 ounces at 6 weeks postpartum.

        - Increased lochia flow and uterine cramping is common during feedings.
        - Lochia transforms from red to pink, and then to white in about 3 weeks.

    - Heavy perspiration and increased urination result from shedding surplus fluids from pregnancy.
    - Many mothers have difficulty urinating, especially those who were catheterized.
    - A mother might not have a bowel movement for a while after birth.
    - A mother who had a cesarean delivery may have gas and temporary bowel dysfunction.

Postpartum Care of Mothers

- Create a relaxed and supportive learning climate that encourages mothers to seek help.
- Help with the first feeding in a noninterfering manner and teach effective positioning and latch.
- Teach feeding behavior and encourage parents to respond to it.
- Keep mothers and babies together and encourage rooming in.

    - Exclusive breastfeeding rates are higher.
    - Mothers recognize feeding behavior and learn to respond to it.
    - The baby's behavior is more responsive.

- Place no restrictions on feedings.
- Help mothers limit interruptions and visitors.
- Help mothers plan rest periods while the baby sleeps.

- Provide effective discharge planning.
- Refer mothers to breastfeeding support groups.

Hyperbilirubinemia (Jaundice)

- Babies are born with large amounts of red blood cells needed for fetal growth.

  - The baby breaks down excess hemoglobin, separates it, and reuses the globin portion.
  - The heme portion transforms to bilirubin; excessive amounts cause jaundice.

- Excessive bilirubin is a health risk to the baby.

  - Unconjugated, unbound bilirubin migrates toward tissues with high fat content.
  - It circulates freely in the bloodstream and can deposit in the brain, skin, muscle tissue, and mucous membranes.
  - It can pass the blood-brain barrier and have a toxic effect on nerve cells in the brain.
  - Prematurity, asphyxia, and hemolytic disease increase the risk.

- Types of jaundice

  - **Physiologic jaundice** is normal newborn jaundice.

    - At birth, a healthy newborn's bilirubin level is 1.5 mg/dl or less.
    - Levels rise to about 6.5 mg/dl by day 3 or 4 and return to less than 1.5 mg/dl by day 10.
    - A bilirubin level below 20 mg/dl is considered safe for a healthy full-term infant.
    - The newborn excretes bilirubin through stooling and passing urine.

  - **Breastfeeding-associated jaundice** results from caloric deprivation and decreased stooling, and responds to increasing the number and quality of breastfeedings.
  - **Breastmilk jaundice** results from an unknown factor present in the mother's milk.

    - It develops at 4 to 7 days of life and peaks by week 2 or 3.
    - It is self-limiting and benign and usually requires no treatment.

  - **Pathologic jaundice** results from infection, disease, obstruction, interference with the binding of bilirubin in the bloodstream, blood incompatibility, and certain drugs.

- Detection of jaundice

  - Jaundice is more frequent among Asians, Native Americans, Eskimos, and babies born at higher altitudes.

  - Jaundice progresses from head to foot:

    - 5 to 7 mg/dl at shoulder level
    - 7 to 10 mg/dl at the umbilicus
    - 10 to 12 mg/dl below the umbilicus
    - 15 mg/dl below the knees

- Treatment of jaundice

  - Increase stooling by increasing effective breastfeeding.
  - Place the baby near a sunny window.
  - Discontinue any drugs that contribute to the buildup of bilirubin.
  - Initiate phototherapy (see Figure 7-1).
  - Perform an exchange transfusion if bilirubin levels do not drop after phototherapy.

Milk Production

Note: See Chapter 9 for problems with milk production.

Establishing Milk Production

- Milk production begins during pregnancy.

  - Colostrum is present from about the fourth month of pregnancy onward.
  - Delivery of the placenta triggers a reduction in progesterone and elevated prolactin.

- Full milk production begins at 3 to 4 days postpartum.

  - Increased blood and lymph in the breast form the nutrients for milk production.
  - The breasts become fuller, heavier, and sometimes tender.
  - A mother who is separated from her baby needs to begin regular milk expression immediately, at least 8 times every 24 hours and once at night when prolactin levels are highest.

- Lactation is established by about 2 to 3 weeks postpartum.

  - The breasts become comfortably soft and pliable and fullness diminishes.
  - Regular, frequent feedings maintain milk production.
  - Avoid missed feedings, especially in the early months.
  - See Chapter 6 for signs of adequate milk intake.

Recommendations for Phototherapy Management

Healthy term newborn ≥ 38 weeks

Age (hours)	Total serum bilirubin level—mgm/dL (μmol/L)	
≤ 24*	—	
25–48	≥ 12 (210)	≥ 15 (260)
49–72	≥ 15 (260)	≥ 17 (310)
>72	≥ 17 (290)	≥ 20 (340)
	Consider phototherapy as a clinical option	Initiate phototherapy

Infants at medium risk ≥ 38 weeks + risk factors or 35–37 6/7 weeks and well

Age (hours)	Total serum bilirubin level—mgm/dL (μmol/L)	
≤ 24*	—	
25–48	≥ 10	≥ 13
49–72	≥ 13	≥ 15
>72	≥ 15	≥ 18
	Initiate phototherapy	Initiate phototherapy

Infants at higher risk 35–37 6/7 weeks + risk factors

Age (hours)	Total serum bilirubin level—mgm/dL (μmol/L)	
≤ 24*	—	
25–48	≥ 8	≥ 11
49–72	≥ 11	≥ 13
>72	≥ 13	≥ 15
	Initiate phototherapy	Initiate phototherapy

*Term infants who are clinically jaundiced at ≤ 24 hours old are not considered healthy and require further evaluation.

Figure 7-1 Recommendations for Phototherapy Management.
Source: Subcommittee on Hyperbilirubinemia. Management of Hyperbilirubinemia in the Newborn Infant 35 or More Weeks of Gestation. *Pediatrics* 114(1); July 2004.

Length of Feeds

- The baby's needs should determine feeding length.

  - Allow the baby to release the breast spontaneously to end the feed.
  - Feedings may be about 15–20 minutes in the early days.
  - A newborn may nurse on only one breast at a feeding and drift off to sleep. As alertness improves, the baby will increase the number of feeds and will feed at both breasts at a session.
  - Limiting time on a breast can prevent the baby from receiving significant hindmilk and result in poor weight gain and coliclike symptoms.
  - As the baby matures and extracts milk efficiently, the time spent at feeds diminishes.

- The baby changes to nonnutritive sucking when milk flow diminishes.

  - The baby's eyes close, the fists relax, and the hands come away from the face.
  - The baby may release the breast and the breast will slide out of the baby's mouth.
  - The mother can switch to the other breast and feed until the baby self-detaches again.

Frequency of Feeds

- The baby's suckling releases **cholecystokinin** (CCK), a gastrointestinal hormone, which enhances digestion, causes sedation, and brings a feeling of satiation and well-being.

  - CCK level peaks immediately after a feed and 30 to 60 minutes later.
  - The baby may arouse to go to the breast not yet nursed between these peaks.

- In the first month, feeding frequency ranges from 8 to 14 feeds daily.

  - Most babies require at least 8 to 10 feeds.
  - Undemanding babies should be aroused to feed after 3 hours.
  - A baby may feed every hour during the day or several times during the night.
  - A baby may cluster some feeds with a longer stretch of sleep.
  - By 8 to 12 weeks of age, a baby feeds every 2 to 3 hours.
  - By around 3 months, the baby drops to 6 or 7 feedings daily.
  - As the baby matures, feeds will be spaced farther apart.

- Feeding frequency increases at several intervals.

  - In the first days at home as the family settles in.

- At around 10 to 14 days (the mother also loses initial breast fullness).
- At around 3 to 6 weeks (the mother's increased activity may cause a drop in milk production).
- At 3 and 6 months, as the baby continues to grow.
- At times of illness, overstimulation, emotional upset, or physical discomfort.

Effective Feeding Practices

Note: See Chapter 9 for problems with positioning and latch.

Observe and Assist at Feedings

- Reinforce feeding behavior, effective positioning, and latch in a noninterfering manner.
- Help cesarean mothers find a comfortable position for nursing.
- Note how the mother holds the baby and whether she needs to hold her breast.
- Note the position of the baby's body, mouth, tongue, head, and hands.

Managing the Feeding

- Put the baby to breast in response to feeding behavior (see Chapter 6) or every 2–3 hours in the early days.
- Help the mother get into a comfortable position with her back supported, using pillows and a footstool as necessary.
- Position the baby in flexion, level with and facing the breast.

  - Cuddle the baby closely around her body.
  - Make sure the baby's ear, shoulder, and hip are in alignment.
  - Place the baby's mouth slightly below the center of the breast to encourage the baby to reach up to the breast.
  - If necessary, pull the baby's lower body in toward the mother with the baby's head angled away from the breast to facilitate breathing.

> **ADVICE TO CLINICIANS**
> **BE ALERT!**
>
> Avoid harmful practices:
>
> ▶ Place no restrictions on feedings.
> ▶ Give supplements only when medically indicated.
> ▶ Never leave formula with a mother without specific instructions.
> ▶ Give no bottles or pacifiers that could limit time at the breast or create nipple preference.
> ▶ Give no water supplementation.
> ▶ Limit unnecessary interventions.
> ▶ Use nipple shields appropriately.

- Support the breast with the thumb on top and fingers curved below, well behind the areola.

  - Angle the nipple up toward the hard palate to help trigger the baby's suck.
  - Tickle the baby's upper lip with the nipple to stimulate the baby's mouth to open wide (see Figure 7-2 and Figure 7-3).

- Bring the baby to the breast quickly when the baby's mouth is open wide.

  - Make sure the baby's lips flange out.
  - The baby's cheeks should be smooth and equidistant from the breast.
  - The baby's tongue should extend over the alveolar ridge.
  - The baby's chin should press into the breast.

- Allow the baby to pace the feeding.

  - The baby should settle into a suck–swallow–breathe pattern of long, deep sucks with one suck per second.
  - Listen for swallowing with no clicking sounds.
  - Break suction if it is necessary to reposition the baby.
  - Insert a finger gently into the corner of the baby's mouth between the gums.
  - The baby will instinctively begin to suck faster when the mother touches the baby's lips.
  - Do not allow the baby to chew or tug on the end of the nipple.
  - Press a finger against the breast near the corner of the baby's mouth.

- Make sure the baby feeds at least 15 to 20 minutes to receive both foremilk and hindmilk.
- Allow the baby to release the breast spontaneously to signal the end of the feed.

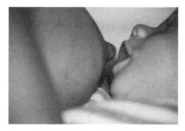

Figure 7-2 Baby's Mouth Beginning to Open. The baby's mouth begins to open; if the mother were to put the baby to breast at this point the baby would not get a good mouthful of breast tissue. Printed with permission of Kay Hoover.

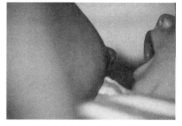

Figure 7-3 Baby's Mouth Open Wide for aGood Latch. The baby's mouth has continued to open wide and the baby is now ready to go to the breast. Printed with permission of Kay Hoover.

Breastfeeding Positions

- **Cradle hold:** The mother sits with the baby's body across her abdomen, rests the baby's head on her forearm and supports the baby's body with her hand (see Figure 7-4).
- **Football (clutch) hold:** The mother holds her baby under her arm along her side with his feet toward her back. She holds the head in her hand, supports the body with her right forearm, and raises the head to breast level (see Figure 7-5).
- **Cross-cradle (dominant hand) position:** The mother rests the baby's head in her hand and supports the body with her forearm. She moves her arm with the baby across her body to the opposite breast (see Figure 7-6).
- **Side-lying position:** The mother lies on her side with her knees slightly bent and her head on a pillow. The baby is placed on his or her side level with and facing the breast, and the mother brings the baby to the breast with her upper arm (see Figure 7-7).
- **Posture feeding (prone position):** The mother lies on her back with her baby tummy to tummy on top of her (see Figure 7-8).

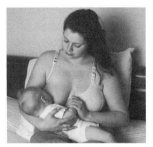

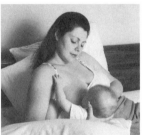

Top to bottom:

Figure 7-4 Cradle Hold Nursing Position

Figure 7-5 Football (Clutch) Nursing Position

Figure 7-6 Cross-Cradle (Dominant Hand) Nursing Position

Figures 7-4 to 7-8 printed with permission of Nelia Box.

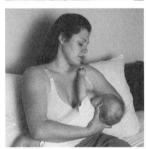

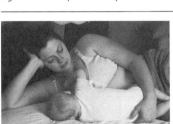

Figure 7-7 Side-Lying Nursing Position

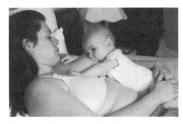

Figure 7-8 Posture Feeding Position

> **ADVICE TO CLINICIANS**
> **EMPOWER STAFF**
>
> ▶ Develop evidence-based breastfeeding policies, and teach healthcare staff how to implement them.
> ▶ Teach physicians correct information about breastfeeding.
> ▶ Promote labor and delivery practices that support early breastfeeding.
> ▶ Limit the use of medications, anesthesia, and other birth interventions.
> ▶ Promote delaying treating the infants' eyes for 1 hour to allow bonding.
> ▶ Teach staff to give supplements only for acceptable medical reasons.
> ▶ Teach staff to give no artificial teats to infants and to use nipple shields appropriately.

Accommodating Special Needs
Multiples

- Breastfeeding multiples:

  - The mother will need pillows and help with positioning her babies (see Figure 7-9).
  - Having babies together for feedings helps the mother learn practical aspects.
  - Breastfeed separately at least one time every day to bond individually.

- Options for feeding twins:

  - Alternate babies between breasts at each feeding, every few feedings, or daily. This ensures equal stimulation of both breasts and coordinated visual development.
  - Place each baby on the same breast at every feed. One baby may have a stronger suck, causing one breast to be larger than the other breast.

- Feeding higher order multiples:

  - Nurse two babies simultaneously while someone feeds the other baby(ies).
  - Nurse two babies simultaneously and the other(s) afterward.
  - Make sure all babies receive the same amount of time at the breast.

- Challenges with multiples:

  - Bonding may be complicated when one baby remains hospitalized longer.
  - Quality of the parents' support system is a large factor in a mother's coping abilities.

- The mother is at risk for mastitis because of fatigue and an abundant milk supply.
- The babies may not be hungry at the same time. Feeding options include:

  ‣ When one baby is hungry, feed both.
  ‣ Delay feeding the hungry baby until the other one will feed.
  ‣ Feed the hungry baby and keep the other one close by to stimulate an interest in feeding.

- The babies will develop and grow at varying rates.

  ‣ Growth spurts may occur at different times.
  ‣ The babies may be ready for complementary foods and weaning at different times.
  ‣ Regard the babies as individuals and meet their separate needs.

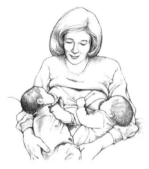

Baby Who Is Too Sleepy to Nurse

- Possible causes of sleepiness:

  - The baby is responding to medications the mother had during labor.
  - The mother had a long labor or long second-stage labor.
  - The baby was born prematurely.
  - It is a usual sleepy period for the baby.
  - The first feeding was delayed.
  - Feeding behavior was overlooked.
  - The baby is experiencing sensory overload, as in a loud nursery.
  - The baby has been crying related to interventions, particularly circumcision.
  - The baby is jaundiced.
  - A schedule has been imposed on feedings.
  - The baby was born by cesarean delivery.
  - The baby is hypothermic.

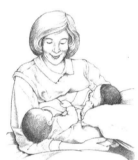

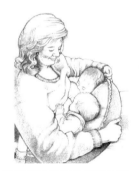

Figure 7-9 Positions for Nursing Multiples
Source: Illustrations by Marcia Smith

- Plan of care for a sleepy baby:

  - Room in with the baby 24 hours/day with skin-to-skin contact.
  - Respond to early feeding behavior.
  - Attempt to put the baby to breast every half hour to hour, when the baby is in a light sleep state.
  - Pump or hand express, and feed the milk to the baby.
  - Monitor the baby's output, and watch for symptoms of dehydration or hypoglycemia.

- Waking a sleepy baby:

  - Talk to the baby, and try to make eye contact.
  - Dim the lights to encourage the baby's eyes to open.
  - Loosen or remove blankets.
  - Hold the baby upright in a sitting or standing position.
  - Partially or fully undress the baby.
  - Change the baby's diaper.
  - Increase skin contact through massage or gently rubbing the baby's hands and feet.
  - Stimulate the baby's rooting reflex.
  - Bring the baby close to the breast to detect the scent of the mother's skin.
  - Express milk onto the nipple or into the baby's mouth to encourage the baby to latch.
  - Wipe the baby's forehead and cheeks with a cool moist cloth.
  - Move the baby's arms and legs.
  - Give the baby a bath or take a bath with the baby for increased skin contact.

- Rousing a baby who latches and does not suck:

  - Stroke under the baby's chin from front to back.
  - Compress the breast as with manual expression.

Baby Who Cries and Resists Going to Breast

- Possible causes of fussiness:

  - Overhandling by caregivers.
  - The baby has or had pain.
  - The mother received medication during labor that passed to the baby.
  - The baby has discomfort from forceps, vacuum extraction, internal monitor lead, or cephalhematoma.
  - The baby has an oral aversion because of deep suctioning or other invasive procedures.
  - The baby is irritable.
  - The baby received an artificial nipple or pacifier, which resulted in nipple preference.

- The mother's lack of confidence causes her to hold her baby tentatively.
- The baby needs to be swaddled to provide boundaries, or soothed by being cuddled skin to skin with the parent.
- The baby has shut down from too much intervention, such as someone attempting to push him or her on the breast.
- The mother and baby were separated, resulting in missed feeding behavior and missed imprinting.
- Rarely, fussiness in a baby can indicate a serious problem, such as a neurological disorder.

- Plan of care for a fussy baby:

  - Hold and cuddle the baby calmly skin to skin at the breast, or swaddle the baby to restrict startling and movement.
  - Use soothing techniques before putting the baby to breast.
  - Begin feedings before the baby becomes too upset or overly hungry.
  - Limit feeding attempts to no more than a few minutes, wait 10 to 15 minutes and try again.
  - Express or pump and feed the milk to the baby.
  - Give no unnecessary bottles or pacifiers.
  - Use calming techniques.

Relactation

- Relactation is reestablishing milk production when production is greatly reduced or has ceased.

  - The baby had an allergic reaction to artificial baby milk.
  - The baby reacted negatively to weaning.
  - The mother weaned prematurely because of misinformation or lack of support.
  - The mother has low milk production because of mismanagement of breastfeeding.
  - The baby rejected the breast or suckled poorly.
  - The mother is experiencing family pressure or guilt from not breastfeeding.

- Factors in success:

  - The degree of breast stimulation and postpartum breast involution:

    - Did the mother begin breastfeeding after birth?
    - How much time elapsed since weaning or birth?

      - Estrogen concentrations fall rapidly immediately after birth.
      - Prolactin levels drop to normal by 3 weeks if not breastfeeding.
      - The degree of breast drainage in the first week determines the number of prolactin receptors.

Calming techniques for a fussy baby:

▶ Limit invasive procedures to minimize crying.
▶ Provide skin-to-skin contact.
▶ Cuddle without pushing the baby to nurse.
▶ Be sensitive to and respond to the baby's behavior.
▶ Build the mother's confidence.
▶ Use slow, calm, deliberate movements in caring for the baby.
▶ Cuddle, hold, and walk with the baby.
▶ Talk or sing to the baby in a soft voice.
▶ Swaddle the baby.
▶ Feed the baby in a dark, quiet room.
▶ Feed in a rocking chair to relax both the mother and baby.
▶ Burp the baby often if it is tolerated. Burp before moving the baby to the other breast.
▶ Carry the baby in a position that puts gentle and firm pressure on the abdomen.
▶ Play music or a monotonous noise.
▶ Change the baby's diaper when it becomes damp or soiled.
▶ Mother and baby sleep or nap together for shared warmth and heartbeat.
▶ Massage the baby for 10 to 15 minutes (the baby may fuss but may become quiet afterward).
▶ Use a sling to carry the baby close to the mother's body.
▶ Use a baby swing for times when individual attention is not possible.
▶ When good temperature control is present, expose the baby to the air for limited amounts of time.
▶ Lay the baby on his or her stomach on the mother's lap and bounce or move the knees back and forth.
▶ Have the mother and baby take a bath together.
▶ Provide monotonous movement with a stroller or car ride.
▶ Remove allergens from the mother's diet.

- How willing is the baby to suckle at the breast?

  ◗ Willingness to suck corresponds to a baby's age, the amount of time away from the breast, and how the baby has been fed.
  ◗ Encourage suckling by simulating birth, with the baby on the mother's abdomen in a bath of warm water.

- Relactation requires that the mother have realistic goals.

  ‣ She is motivated and committed; she, not the caregiver, should initiate the topic.
  ‣ She will adjust her lifestyle to give total attention to relactation.
  ‣ She has support or she can proceed without support.
  ‣ She avoids milk-reducing influences such as oral contraceptives, nicotine, and herbal teas such as peppermint and sage.
  ‣ She measures success in terms of bonding rather than the amount of milk or length of breastfeeding.

- Managing relactation:

  - Create a relaxed atmosphere without pressure to nurse.
  - Provide frequent and continuous skin-to-skin contact.
  - Attempt feeds when the baby is drowsy or in a light sleep state.
  - Massage the breast before beginning the feeding to make milk available.
  - Drip breastmilk or formula on the end of the nipple to encourage suckling.
  - Alternate between breasts several times during a feeding.
  - Pump with a double electric breast pump.

    ‣ In the absence of suckling, match frequency to the baby's feeding pattern.
    ‣ Pump between feedings to supplement nipple stimulation.

  - Supplement the baby at the breast with a tube-feeding device.

    ‣ Supplement with donor milk or artificial baby milk until full production is achieved.
    ‣ Decrease the amount of supplement in response to increased milk production.
    ‣ Work closely with the baby's caregiver and monitor the baby's weight.

Adopted Baby

- Inducing lactation in the absence of pregnancy is challenging.

  - The mother needs realistic motives and expectations, as with relactation.
  - The woman lacks the estrogen concentrations that occur during pregnancy that prepare the breasts for lactation.
  - Prolactin levels may not sufficiently stimulate milk secretion.

    ‣ If the woman has been pregnant, she is three times as likely to have milky secretions.
    ‣ If a hormonal imbalance prevented pregnancy, the imbalance could affect lactation.

- Prepare for breastfeeding before placement.

  - Check for inverted nipples, and avoid soap and other drying agents.
  - Massage the breasts 5–8 times daily over 3–6 months.
  - Pump with a hospital-grade double electric breast pump up to 1 month before placement, every 2–3 hours during the day for 10 minutes.
  - Attend a support group for breastfeeding or adoptive nursing women.
  - Request that caregivers not use a bottle to feed the baby.
  - Request the opportunity to breastfeed after the birth.

- Managing induced lactation:

  - Use the same techniques as for relactation.
  - Milk production will increase more rapidly after the baby begins suckling.

    - Babies younger than 3 months are more likely to suckle.
    - Keep the baby in bed with the mother to increase suckling.
    - Milk quantity will increase much more slowly than that of a biologic mother.

  - Supplement with donor milk or artificial baby milk.

    - Milk of adoptive mothers is not adequate as total nourishment.
    - Keep a diary of supplemental feedings and breastfeedings.
    - Decrease supplements slowly, not exceeding 25 ml per feeding.
    - Monitor the baby's growth and output for 4 to 7 days before another decrease.

  - Visit the baby's caregiver for frequent weight checks and signs of growth.

Postpartum Care Plans
48-Hour Hospital Stay

- Labor and delivery:

  - Teach how to position the baby for the first feeding.
  - Teach feeding behavior the baby exhibits.
  - Keep the baby skin-to-skin with the mother.
  - Keep the room quiet, with dim lights and low stimulation.
  - Delay visitors for the first hour.

- Hours 1–8:

  - Observe a feeding; there is usually at least one feed in the first 8 hours.
  - Reinforce positioning and latch.
  - Teach the difference between nutritive and nonnutritive sucking.
  - Reinforce feeding behavior and putting the baby to breast according to behavior.
  - Keep the baby and mother together.

- Hours 9–16:

  - The baby should nurse 2 or more times.
  - If the baby has not nursed by 10 to 12 hours, begin pumping or expressing milk.
  - If the baby is not latching, feed expressed milk.
  - Review risk factors for problems and take appropriate action (see Figure 7-10 and Figure 7-11).

- Hours 17–24:

  - The baby should nurse two or more times, for at least six feedings in the first 24 hours.
  - The mother should be able to demonstrate effective positioning and latch.
  - Observe a feeding and ask the mother to point out nutritive and nonnutritive sucking.
  - If the baby is still not latching, continue to express milk and feed to the baby and refer to an IBCLC.

Red Flags and Risk Factors for Breastfeeding Problems

Maternal Factors

- Gained less than 18 pounds during pregnancy
- Previous breast surgery or breast trauma
- Little or no change in breast size or color during pregnancy
- History of low milk supply or breastfeeding "failure" with previous infants
- History of hypothyroidism, infertility, polycystic ovarian syndrome (PCOS), or other androgen or endocrine disorder
- Hypoplasia of the breasts
- Flat or inverted nipples or taut, tight breast tissue
- Primipara
- Gestational diabetes or diabetic (either oral or insulin dependent)
- Epidural in labor
  - In place longer than 3–4 hours before delivery
  - Put in more than one time
  - Received more than 1 bolus of epidural medication
- Induction of labor with Pitocin
- Received excessive intravenous fluids; on magnesium sulfate; postdelivery edema newly present in ankles
- Pain medication for labor more than 1 hour prior to delivery
- Had a cesarean delivery
- Breastfeeding initiated more than 1 hour after delivery
- Sore nipples throughout a feeding at the time of hospital discharge

Figure 7-10 Maternal Risk Factors in Breastfeeding.
Source: Lactation Education Consultants. Printed with permission of Jan Barger and Linda Kutner.

Red Flags and Risk Factors for Breastfeeding Problems

Infant Factors

- Less than 38 weeks gestation
- Weighs less than 7 pounds
- Male infant
- Vacuum or forceps used for delivery
- Infant has ankyloglossia (tight frenulum) or cleft lip or palate or both
- Fetal distress; meconium release during delivery
- Insult to the oral cavity (laryngoscope and deep suctioning)
- The infant is kept in the nursery instead of with the mother
- SGA (small for gestational age) or LGA (large for gestational age)
- Feeding restrictions placed on the infant (timed feedings, NPO)
- Multiple bottles given during hospitalization
- Use of a pacifier more than 30 minutes per day
- Jaundice
- The infant is sleepy, difficult to wake; fails to demonstrate clear feeding behavior
- Difficulty latching on consistently; has not established effective breastfeeding by hospital discharge
- 7% or greater weight loss at time of hospital discharge

All factors can contribute to problems with breastfeeding. Some are more significant than others. Multiple factors indicate that the dyad *must* be followed after discharge from hospital. The goal of this list is to identify potential dyads that may have problems establishing either an adequate milk supply or positive milk transfer. The health worker can work with them while they overcome their problems, in a manner that is both safe and supportive of the breastfeeding experience.

Figure 7-11 Infant Risk Factors in Breastfeeding.
Source: Lactation Education Consultants. Printed with permission of Jan Barger and Linda Kutner.

- Hours 25–32:

  - The baby should nurse two or more times.
  - Reinforce the number of feedings, wet diapers, and stools needed in a 24-hour period.
  - Give the mother a breastfeeding diary.
  - Teach the mother how to know when breastfeeding is going well (see Figure 7-12).
  - Teach warning signs that indicate a problem and when to call an IBCLC.
  - Teach how to prevent nipple soreness and engorgement.

Signs That Breastfeeding Is Going Well

Breastfeeding is going well if:

- The baby is nursing at least eight times in 24 hours.
- The baby has at least six wet and three soiled diapers every 24 hours.
- The mother can hear her baby gulping or swallowing at feeds.
- The breasts feel softer after a feed.
- The mother's nipples are not painful, and breastfeeding is enjoyable.

The mother may need help if:

- The baby has fewer than six wet diapers daily after day 4.
- The baby still has meconium or fewer than three soiled diapers daily after day 4.
- The breasts feel full, but the mother cannot hear her baby gulping or swallowing.
- The mother's nipples are painful throughout the feeding.
- The baby seems to be nursing all the time.
- The mother does not feel her milk production is full after day 4.
- The baby is gaining less than ½ ounce daily or has not regained birth weight by 10 days of age.

Figure 7-12 Signs That Breastfeeding Is Going Well

- Hours 33–40:

    - Observe and document a complete feeding, with the mother positioning and latching the baby on unassisted.
    - Recommend a normal healthy diet and drinking when thirsty.
    - Teach about cluster feedings, role of the father, avoidance of artificial nipples, risks of artificial baby milk, cosleeping, and anticipatory guidance for the first few nights home.

- Hours 41–48:

    - The baby should be latching on and nursing well before leaving the hospital.
    - The mother should observe nutritive sucking and swallowing during feedings.
    - The mother should appear comfortable holding, dressing, and diapering the baby.
    - Teach that feeding behavior is in place 20 to 30 minutes before sustained crying and that crying compromises and disorganizes a baby's suck.

- Discharge:

    - Teach signs of adequate milk production.
    - Provide information on community resources and breast pumps.
    - Confirm when the baby will be checked for weight and skin color.

24-Hour Hospital Stay

- Labor and delivery:

    - Teach how to position the baby for the first feeding.
    - Teach feeding behavior the baby exhibits.
    - Keep the baby skin-to-skin with the mother.
    - Keep the room quiet, with dim lights and low stimulation.
    - Delay visitors for the first hour.

- Hours 1–8:

    - Observe a feeding; there is usually at least one feed in the first 8 hours.
    - Reinforce feeding behavior and putting the baby to breast according to behavior.
    - Reinforce positioning and latch.
    - Teach the difference between nutritive and nonnutritive sucking.
    - Keep the baby and mother together.
    - Reinforce the number of feedings, wet diapers, and stools needed in a 24-hour period.
    - Give the mother a breastfeeding diary.
    - Teach how to know when breastfeeding is going well.
    - Teach warning signs that indicate a problem.

- Hours 9–16:

    - The baby should nurse two or more times.
    - If the baby has not nursed by 10 to 12 hours, begin pumping or expressing milk.
    - If the baby is not latching, feed expressed milk.
    - Review the risk factors for problems and take appropriate action.

- Hours 17–24:

    - The baby should nurse two or more times, for at least six feedings in the first 24 hours.
    - Observe a feeding, and ask the mother to point out nutritive and nonnutritive sucking.
    - The mother should be able to demonstrate effective positioning and latch.
    - The baby should be latching on and nursing well before leaving the hospital.

        ▶ If the baby is still not latching by the middle of this shift:

            – Delay discharge until the baby has at least two effective feeds.
            – Continue to express milk and feed to the baby until effective feeds are established.
            – Refer the mother to an IBCLC to develop a feeding plan.

▶ When the baby is latching well:

  – Recommend a normal healthy diet and drinking when thirsty.
  – Teach how to prevent nipple soreness and engorgement.
  – Teach when to call an IBCLC.
  – Teach that feeding behavior is in place 20 to 30 minutes before sustained crying and that crying compromises and disorganizes a baby's suck.

• Discharge:

  ▪ Teach signs of adequate milk production.
  ▪ Provide information on community resources and breast pumps.
  ▪ Confirm when the baby will be checked for weight and skin color.

Tutorial for Students and Interns

Key Clinical Management Strategies

From *Clinical Guidelines for the Establishment of Exclusive Breastfeeding*, ILCA, 2005.

• Assess the mother and infant for signs of effective breastfeeding and intervene if breastfeeding is ineffective.
• Assist the mother and infant in achieving a comfortable position and effective latch (attachment).
• Confirm that mothers understand normal breastfed infant behaviors and have realistic expectations regarding infant care and breastfeeding.
• Observe and document at least one breastfeeding in each 8-hour period during the postpartum period.
• Teach mothers to recognize and respond to early infant feeding cues and confirm that the baby is being fed at least eight times in each 24 hours.
• Confirm that mothers recognize how to wake a sleepy infant.
• Confirm that mothers understand the physiology of milk production, especially the role of milk removal.
• Confirm that the infant has a scheduled appointment with a primary care provider or health worker within 5 to 7 days after birth.
• Facilitate breastfeeding within the first hour after birth and provide for continuous skin-to-skin contact between mother and infant until after the first feeding.
• Keep the mother and infant together during the entire postpartum stay.
• Provide appropriate breastfeeding education materials.
• Avoid using pacifiers, artificial nipples, and supplements, unless medically indicated.

Key Clinical Competencies

From *Clinical Competencies for IBCLC Practice* available at www.iblce.org.

- ☐ Perform a comprehensive breastfeeding assessment.
- ☐ Assess and evaluate the infant's ability to breastfeed.
- ☐ Assess effective milk transfer.
- ☐ Evaluate effectiveness of the breastfeeding plan.
- ☐ Identify events that occurred during the labor and birth process that may negatively impact breastfeeding.
- ☐ Identify and discourage practices that may interfere with breastfeeding.
- ☐ Identify correct latch (attachment).
- ☐ Develop a breastfeeding risk assessment.
- ☐ Develop an appropriate breastfeeding plan in concert with the mother.
- ☐ Observe a feeding.
- ☐ Promote continuous skin-to-skin contact of the term newborn and mother until the first feeding.
- ☐ Help the mother and infant to find a comfortable position for latching (attachment) during the initial feeding after birth.
- ☐ Assist the mother and family to identify newborn feeding cues.
- ☐ Assist mothers with cesarean birth.
- ☐ Assist mothers with traumatic birth.
- ☐ Assist mothers with infants born at 35–38 weeks gestation.
- ☐ Assist mothers with infants that are small or large for gestational age.
- ☐ Assist mothers with preterm birth, including the benefits of kangaroo care.
- ☐ Assist mothers with multiples or plural births.
- ☐ Assist mothers with flat or inverted nipples.
- ☐ Assist mothers with maintaining milk production.
- ☐ Assist mothers with increasing milk production.
- ☐ Assist mothers with sleepy infants.
- ☐ Assist mothers with infants who have hyperbilirubinemia (jaundice).
- ☐ Assist mothers with induced lactation and relactation.
- ☐ Assist mothers with cultural beliefs that are not evidence-based and may interfere with breastfeeding (e.g., discarding colostrum, rigidly scheduled feedings, necessity of artificial baby milk after every breastfeeding).
- ☐ Assist mothers with care of their breasts.
- ☐ Assist mothers with infants at high risk for hypoglycemia.
- ☐ Assist mothers with continuation of breastfeeding when the mother is separated from her baby.
- ☐ Assist mothers with milk expression techniques.
- ☐ Reinforce keeping the mother and baby together.
- ☐ Reinforce feeding the baby on cue—but at least eight times in each 24-hour period.
- ☐ Instruct the mother about avoidance of the early use of a pacifier and bottle nipple.
- ☐ Instruct the mother about plans for follow-up care for breastfeeding questions, infant's medical, and mother's postpartum examinations.

☐ Instruct the mother about normal newborn behavior, including why, when, and how to wake a sleepy newborn.

☐ Instruct the mother about how milk is produced and supply maintained, including discussion of growth and appetite spurts.

☐ Instruct the mother about prevention and treatment of sore nipples.

☐ Instruct the mother about prevention and treatment of engorgement.

☐ Instruct the mother about assessment of adequate milk intake by the baby.

☐ Instruct the mother about normal infant sucking patterns.

☐ Use appropriate resources for research to provide information to the healthcare team on conditions and medications that affect breastfeeding and lactation.

From Theory to Practice
Birth and Postpartum Care

1. What can labor and delivery staff do immediately after delivery to optimize breastfeeding for a mother and her infant?

2. You are asked to help update your hospital protocol for laboring women. What items will you include in the protocol to protect breastfeeding?

3. Bonding, rooting, and sucking are particularly strong in the first 2 hours after birth. How will you respond to a mother who is upset that she missed that opportunity because she and her baby were separated for the first 4 hours?

4. How does breastfeeding help the mother's uterus return to its prepregnant state?

5. A mother tells you she wants her baby kept in the nursery during the night so she can get a good night's sleep. What can you say to encourage her to room in with her baby?

6. At 24 hours of age, a newborn has not yet had a good feeding. It has been 3 hours since the mother last attempted a feed. When you enter her room, she is visiting with several friends and relatives. She tells you she will nurse again when she is finished visiting. How will you respond?

7. A young mother has just learned that her baby cannot be discharged with her because he must receive phototherapy in the special care unit for the next 24 hours. She asks you what she did wrong to cause her baby's bilirubin level to get so high. How will you respond to her?

8. What hospital practices will help to minimize the possibility of jaundice in a newborn?

9. What are the health implications of breastmilk, physiologic, and pathologic jaundice?

10. At 3 days of life, a newborn's skin coloring has a yellowish tinge that extends to the knees. What is the recommendation for phototherapy management?

11. What counseling approach can help parents of a jaundiced baby avoid viewing their baby as vulnerable to illness?

12. How soon and how often does a mother need to express her milk if she is unable to begin nursing immediately after birth because her baby aspirated meconium during delivery?

13. What are the potential consequences of failing to initiate breastfeeding immediately after delivery?
14. A mother returned from her baby's 1-week visit to the pediatrician and tells you her baby suddenly developed jaundice and she has to wean. How would you approach helping her? What would be your first statement to her?

Milk Production

15. Describe what happens at the time of delivery that triggers milk production.
16. What happens to the mother's breasts when lactation becomes well established?
17. Why is it important to allow the baby to determine the length of a feed?
18. How does cholecystokinin affect the baby?
19. How does the length of feeds change as the baby matures?
20. What are the signs that the baby is ready to end a feed?
21. What feeding frequency can a mother expect in the first month?
22. How does a baby's feeding frequency change during the 3rd and 4th month?
23. What causes a baby to alter feeding frequency in the first days home?
24. How should a mother respond to growth spurts?
25. Realizing you need to limit suggestions to three or four, what would you teach mothers about how to tell they have sufficient milk?

Breastfeeding Assistance

26. How can you teach and reinforce effective positioning and latch in a noninterfering manner?
27. A mother is unable to sit or turn her body immediately after delivery. How can you help her initiate breastfeeding?
28. How would you help a mother who delivered by cesarean section and is having difficulty getting comfortable for feedings?
29. What feeding plan will you recommend for a mother who is unable to begin breastfeeding her baby during the first 24 hours after birth?
30. What are all the elements of the placement of the baby's mouth that need to be observed at a feeding?
31. In which ways does a baby self-regulate feeds?
32. How is a footstool helpful in positioning for a feed?
33. Why might a mother have difficulty positioning her baby for a good latch when she holds her baby in the cradle position?
34. When is it appropriate for a mother to break suction to remove her baby from the breast?

Accommodating a Baby's Needs

35. What feeding plan would you recommend to a mother who can take only one of her twins home at discharge while the other twin remains in the hospital for the next week?

36. How can a mother of twins make sure she receives equal stimulation to both breasts?

37. Why would a loud nursery cause a baby to be sleepy?

38. A 2-day-old baby is too sleepy to nurse effectively. Keeping in mind that you want to limit the number of suggestions you give to a mother at one time, what will you suggest to encourage her baby to nurse?

39. How would you help a mother who is concerned that her 2-day-old baby falls asleep after 15 minutes on one breast and does not nurse on the other breast?

40. A mother's 2-day-old baby sucks intermittently but sleeps for most of the time at the breast. How can she increase her baby's effectiveness at the breast?

41. A mother's 2-day-old baby cries every time she attempts to nurse. What might cause the fussiness, and how can you help her at a feeding?

42. What can the mother of a fussy baby do to prepare for feedings?

43. The mother of a newborn has two children at home, aged 2 and 3 years. Her newborn is fussy and she spends a great deal of time trying to settle her baby into feeds in the hospital. She asks how she can handle feedings after she is home and caring for her other two children. How do you respond?

44. The mother of a 2-week-old infant has been supplementing with artificial baby milk and her milk production is minimal. She wishes to increase production so that she can breastfeed exclusively. What are her chances of reaching that goal and how can you help her?

45. How can remedial cobathing help a mother who is attempting to relactate?

Care Plans

46. Which teaching points in the 48-hour discharge plan are omitted in the 24-hour discharge plan? How can you make sure a mother who is scheduled for a 24-hour discharge leaves with appropriate teaching?

47. What pattern of feeds do you want to see in each 8-hour period of the first 24 hours?

48. What will you recommend to a mother whose baby has not had a good feed by 20 hours? How will you alter this recommendation if the mother is scheduled for a 24-hour discharge?

49. What will you recommend to a mother whose baby has had only two feeds by 16 hours?

50. Based on the 48-hour care plan, how many total feeds should a baby have before discharge?

CHAPTER 8

High-Risk Infants

In This Chapter

Prolonged Hospitalization

Parents' Reactions to Having a High-Risk Infant

- The neonatal intensive care unit (NICU) environment can be unsettling to parents.
- It may be difficult to absorb and process information; repeat, review, and clarify important points.
- Parents experience feelings of detachment, grief, guilt, loneliness, and anxiety.
- Parents grieve if their baby must be transferred to another facility.
- Parents will have pressure from other demands.
- Worry about the baby's condition may cause problems to surface in their relationship.

  - Encourage support within the hospital, the family, and the community.
  - Focus on the mother rather than on her baby.

The Neonatal Intensive Care Unit (NICU)

- There are three levels of NICUs:

  - A level I unit provides routine newborn care.
  - A level II unit cares for newborns that require monitoring and special newborn care.

- A level III unit is a high-risk facility equipped to care for the smallest and sickest babies.

- Care of the high-risk baby in the NICU:

  - Most contact is technical or medical in nature.
  - Feeding may begin with intravenous amino acids, glucose, electrolytes, and vitamins.
  - Gavage feeding via nasogastric tubing may cause an oral aversion.
  - Encourage interaction between parents and baby, with privacy and time alone.

Kangaroo Care

- Kangaroo care can begin as soon as the baby's condition permits, even when on a ventilator.

  - Place the baby skin-to-skin, upright and prone, between the mother's breasts, wearing only a diaper.
  - Wrap the mother and baby together to maintain the baby's temperature adequately.
  - The mother sits quietly with minimal or no sound or movement.
  - The baby may be in a quiet alert state initially and then settle down to sleep.
  - Fathers are encouraged to kangaroo their baby as well as the mother.

- Benefits of kangaroo care:

  - Kangaroo care may assist in recovery from respiratory distress.
  - The baby cries less, has more regular heart rate and respirations, and sleeps better.
  - Heart, respiratory, temperature, and oxygen saturation rates remain stable.
  - Babies tend to gain weight faster and leave the hospital earlier.
  - Kangaroo care prevents neonatal hypothermia in most developing countries.
  - Neonatal pain from heel sticks diminishes when the baby is held skin to skin.
  - Mothers feel more attached to their babies and more confident in caring for them.

ADVICE TO CLINICIANS
BE EMPOWERING

Teach parents of a high-risk infant to do the following:

▶ Ask the baby's caregivers for explanations and clarification.

▶ Continue close medical supervision of the baby until no longer needed.

▶ Monitor the baby's intake, output, and weight.

▶ Base expectations on gestational age rather than on age from birth.

▶ Provide gentle, warm, loving touch to the baby.

▶ Use gentle waking techniques and plenty of skin-to-skin contact.

▶ Participate in feeding, bathing, and diapering.

- Parental participation increases in caring for and comforting their baby.
- The baby becomes familiar with the feeding environment and explores feeding.
- Lying quietly by the breast gradually develops into rooting, licking, and tasting.
- Milk production may improve.

Taking the High-Risk Baby Home

- The baby must demonstrate readiness for discharge.

  - The baby must be physically stable and able to maintain body temperature.
  - The baby must be able to suck on a bottle nipple or breast and tolerate feedings by mouth.

- Parents may feel anxious and overwhelmed with the thought of caring for the baby full time.

  - Refer them to resources such as home health, specialized day care providers, respite caregivers, WIC, Medicaid, and other social services.
  - The mother must initiate and maintain milk production after a delay in breastfeeding and in the absence of feeding behavior.
  - Parents may worry about their baby's survival and react to their baby's breathing noises, spitting up, and behavior.
  - Feelings of guilt, loneliness, and anxiety may strain the couple's relationship.

The Preterm Infant
Profile of a Preterm Infant

- Description:

  - There are three types of preterm intrauterine growth.

    - A baby appropriate for gestational age (AGA) has a normal rate of intrauterine growth.
    - A baby with intrauterine growth retardation (IUGR) has slowed intrauterine growth.
    - Birth weight of a baby born small for gestational age (SGA) is below the 10th percentile.

  - A preterm infant is born before 37 weeks of gestation with a birth weight less than 5½ pounds (2500 g).
  - Skin is loose and wrinkled, with a gelatinous appearance.
  - Blood vessels and bony structures are visible because of little subcutaneous fat.
  - Fine downy hairs may be present on the sides of the face, forehead, back, and extremities.

- There is scant hair on the head, and usually absent eyebrows.
- Cartilage needed to support the ears is underdeveloped, causing the ears to fold.
- The head appears large in proportion to the rest of the body.

- Health challenges:

  - The lungs and rib cage may not function efficiently at birth due to muscular weakness.
  - Heat regulation is poorly developed.
  - Immature liver and digestive systems and low levels of glucuronic acid increase the incidence of physiologic jaundice.
  - Common problems for SGA infants:

    - Regulation of blood sugar and body temperature
    - Ineffective breastfeeding and need for supplementation
    - The need for frequent feedings, as if trying to gain weight not gained in utero

  - The baby's crying behavior varies according to gestational age.

    - Cries of a preterm infant may be more frequent, high pitched, and uneven than those of a full-term baby.
    - More preterm babies develop coliclike symptoms than do full-term babies.

Human Milk for the Preterm Infant

- Human milk may be vital to the progress of a high-risk infant at risk for infection.

  - It establishes enteral tolerance and allows for earlier discontinuation of parenteral nutrition.
  - It has a positive effect on direct and indirect bilirubin levels.
  - Long-term neurodevelopment improves.
  - The protein balance is ideal for babies weighing 1500 grams or more.
  - Babies below 1500 grams need increased calories, carbohydrates, and proteins.

- Human milk fortifiers improve short-term weight gain and linear and head growth.

  - They provide protein, calcium, potassium phosphate, carbohydrates, vitamins, and trace minerals.
  - Data is insufficient to evaluate long-term neurodevelopmental and growth outcomes.
  - VLBW babies need more calcium, phosphorus, and fat-soluble vitamins.

- Lactoengineering provides increased calories, carbohydrates, and proteins.

  - Creamatocrits estimate the fat and energy content of milk.
  - Hindmilk that rises to the top is skimmed off and given to the baby, increasing fat intake.
  - Human milk is the feeding of choice to promote neurodevelopment.

- Preserve the safety of expressed milk.

  - Practice good hygiene when pumping milk.
  - Boil pump parts daily, rinse immediately with cold water after use, and wash in hot soapy water.
  - Store milk in sterile hard plastic or glass containers.
  - Store milk from each pumping separately and label it according to hospital specifications.

- Learn how the hospital wishes to receive expressed milk.

  - Composition of freshly expressed milk is most suitable for the baby.
  - Frozen milk loses some of its protective properties but is preferable to artificial substitutes.
  - Wrap milk in paper or a towel and transport it in a cold insulated container to avoid thawing.

- Feeding expressed milk:

  - Initial feedings are often via nasogastric or orogastric gavage tubing.
  - A gastrostomy tube may be placed through the skin directly into the stomach.
  - Until able to suck nutritively at the breast, the baby can suckle on a drained breast.

    ▸ The baby can practice coordinating a pattern of suck–swallow–breathe.
    ▸ The baby learns to associate the breast with the smell of the mother's milk.

  - Oral feedings begin when the baby stabilizes and can tolerate enteral feedings.
  - Bottle feeding is associated with hypoxemia, hypoxia, hypercapnia, apnea, bradycardia, and cyanosis.

Establishing Milk Production

- Begin to express milk within 6 hours of the baby's birth.

  - Pump at least eight times every 24 hours for 10 to 15 minutes.
  - Include a session during the late evening or early morning.

- Increase the amount of expressed milk as needed.

  - Massage before and during pumping sessions.
  - Pump more frequently. Longer pumping sessions do not increase milk yield.
  - Frequent pumping in the early weeks determines the amount produced long term.

- Stimulating milk release:

  - Provide sensory stimulation with the baby's picture or the smell of the baby's clothing.
  - Provide auditory and visual relaxation.
  - Massage the mother's back while she is pumping.
  - Use galactogogues such as fenugreek or blessed thistle.
  - Use prescription medications such as metoclopramide or domperidone.

- Milk production can fluctuate.

  - Production may fluctuate in response to the baby's condition or changes in lifestyle.
  - Returning to work while the baby remains in the NICU may decrease production.
  - A decrease in production or delay in milk ejection may be unexplained.
  - A mother may produce more milk than the baby is able to use.

Breastfeeding the Preterm Infant

- Readiness to breastfeed:

  - A baby is ready when stable and able to coordinate sucking and swallowing with only occasional disruptions in breathing and heart rate.

    - Babies as young as 30 weeks gestation and as small as 1100 grams can breastfeed.
    - It is easier to suckle on the human breast than with an artificial nipple.
    - A preterm infant can suckle well enough at the breast to achieve good weight gain.

  - Readiness is not dependent on the baby's size or ability to suck on a bottle.

    - Oxygen desaturation is lower during breastfeeding.
    - There are fewer episodes of apnea and bradycardia with breastfeeding.
    - Size does not correlate with ability to coordinate sucking, swallowing, and breathing.
    - Sucking motions and swallowing of amniotic fluid occur early in gestation.

- Transitioning to breastfeeding:

  - Condition the baby to breastfeed.

    ▶ Express milk onto a breast pad and place it near the baby.
    ▶ Place a picture of the mother in the baby's view.
    ▶ Insert a gavage tube through a bottle nipple.
    ▶ Provide frequent skin contact.
    ▶ Conduct practice sessions at the breast.
    ▶ Shape and hold the breast for the baby with the Dancer hand position.
    ▶ Express milk into the baby's mouth.
    ▶ Supplement with a tube-feeding device at feedings.

  - The first breastfeeding usually occurs in the hospital as the baby's condition improves.

    ▶ The mother may feel stressed and awkward and doubt her milk production.
    ▶ The baby may have a poor sucking reflex or be confused about how to suckle.
    ▶ The baby may appear disinterested in breastfeeding.

  - Plan for relaxed and unhurried feedings.

    ▶ Expect minimal feeding interspersed with frequent resting times.
    ▶ Minimize stimulation from bright lights, loud noises, stroking, rocking, or talking.
    ▶ Comfort the baby at the breast with kangaroo care.
    ▶ Hold the baby level with the breast and support the baby's entire body.
    ▶ The football or cross cradle position enables optimal control.
    ▶ The Dancer hand position supports the baby's jaw, minimizes the weight of the breast in the baby's mouth, and helps increase milk intake.
    ▶ Breast massage before and during the feeding encourages the baby to nurse.
    ▶ Express milk to initiate milk flow.

ADVICE TO CLINICIANS
TEACH PARENTS

Feeding tips for high-risk infants:

▶ Express milk to maintain milk production and to stimulate milk release.
▶ Watch closely for subtle feeding behavior.
▶ Plan for unhurried, long, frequent feedings with long periods of rest.
▶ Watch for responses that show signs of overstimulation.
▶ Support the baby's jaw with the Dancer hand position, and help the baby open his or her mouth.
▶ Go no longer than 3 hours between feedings during the day.
▶ Encourage nonnutritive sucking on a drained breast.
▶ Use a nipple shield as necessary.

HIGH-RISK INFANTS

- The baby may experience gulping and choking.

  - Hold the baby so the back of his or her throat is higher than the breast.
  - Sit in a semireclined position.
  - Express milk before the feeding so milk flow is less intense.

Taking the Preterm Infant Home

- Rooming in for several days before discharge allows the mother to function independently with help available if needed.

- Refer the mother to a lactation consultant.

- Age and weight parameters:

  - Preterm infants usually leave the hospital when they reach 35 weeks gestational age.
  - Infants as small as 3½ pounds (1600 grams) may go home when they are doing well.
  - An infant less than 3 pounds (1350 grams) with serious respiratory, heart, or brain problems, or other medical complications usually remains hospitalized.

- Other requirements for discharge:

  - A good sucking reflex
  - Few respiratory problems
  - No signs of disease or complications
  - Good weight gain

- Breastfeeding at home:

  - Continue hospital routines for the first few days to ease the transition to home.
  - Continue expressing milk until the baby breastfeeds more frequently and more efficiently.
  - Discontinue any supplements gradually.
  - Achieving exclusive breastfeeding may take several days or months.

    - The mother may need to increase milk production.
    - The mother may need to adjust to her baby's sucking pattern after pumping.
    - Continue pumping if unable to breastfeed every 2 or 3 hours.
    - Supplement if the baby nurses frequently and does not transfer milk adequately.

  - Monitor intake and weight as feeding routines change.

- Learn how to identify a pattern of nutritive, high-flow sucks and swallows.
- A tube-feeding device may encourage more effective sucking at the breast.
- The baby may need supplementary feedings for increased calories.
- Test weights will monitor milk intake in order to calculate supplement needs.

- Follow up with the mother.

    - Feeding behavior is not always evident with preterm infants.
    - It may take up to 2 years to reach the developmental state of a full-term baby of the same age. Base expectations on the baby's gestational age rather than age from birth.
    - Protect the baby from illness and other conditions that could compromise his or her health.
    - Supervise progress closely, particularly when medical problems are evident.

- Mothers who return to bottle feeding:

    - Caregivers strongly urge mothers to breastfeed their ill babies.
    - Those who had not planned to breastfeed may switch to bottle feeding.
    - Support the mother and help her wean.

The Late Preterm Infant
Profile of a Late Preterm Infant

- A healthy infant born at 35 to 38 weeks
- Generally able to maintain body temperature
- Weighs at or above 2500 grams
- Seems to breastfeed well in the hospital
- Appears healthy and competent
- At risk for readmission to the hospital due to jaundice or weight loss

Breastfeeding Problems After Discharge

- Cardiorespiratory instability can cause the baby to tire quickly.
- The baby can have poor temperature control and metabolic instability.
- The rooting reflex can be immature.
- The suck–swallow–breathe cycle can be uncoordinated.
- Immature oromotor development results in underdeveloped buccal fat pads and masseter muscles.
- Low muscle tone makes it difficult to draw in the nipple, maintain latch, and compress the nipple.
- The mother's nipple may be too large for the baby's small mouth.

Behavior Characteristics

- The baby can go quickly from a hyperalert state to deep sleep.
- The baby demonstrates very subtle feeding behavior or none at all.
- The baby has difficulty tuning out excessive stimulation.
- Decreased albumin sites can make the baby sleepy and at increased risk for jaundice.
- When the original due date arrives, the baby will typically "wake up" and begin to breastfeed.

Breastfeeding Precautions

- Ensure adequate feeding frequency.

  - Make sure the baby nurses at least eight times in 24 hours.
  - Shorter, more frequent feedings may prevent the baby from tiring at the breast.
  - Go no longer than 3 hours between feedings during the day, with a 4-hour stretch at night.
  - Watch closely for subtle feeding behavior, and breastfeed as often as the baby indicates a need.
  - Use gentle waking techniques and plenty of skin-to-skin contact.

- Help the mother initiate and maintain milk production.

  - Express milk until the original due date approaches or until the baby is well over birth weight and milk production is established.
  - Double pump four times a day for 10 to 15 minutes with a hospital-grade pump.
  - Monitor weight with weekly weight checks.
  - A nipple shield may help the baby transfer milk.

The Postterm Infant

Profile of a Postterm Infant

- Birth date is after 42 weeks gestation.
- Body length may be appropriate for gestational age.
- Weight is often small-for-date because of placental deterioration.
- Skin is dry, cracked, sagging and loose, with an absence of vernix.
- Scalp hair is profuse.
- Nails on the fingers and toes are long.

Delivery and Postpartum Care

- Birth may be through induction of labor or cesarean section.
- Fetal oxygenation will be marginal or depressed before labor.
- Meconium may secrete during labor, causing yellow-green staining of the baby's skin and nails.
- Maintaining respiration, blood sugar levels, and nervous functioning may be difficult.
- Initial attempts at breastfeeding will be sluggish, requiring coaxing and prodding.
- Feeding behavior matures as the baby gains weight.

Infant Loss
When a Baby Dies

- Ask her baby's name and use it during your discussion; this acknowledges her baby's importance.
- Let the mother know how saddened you feel, and encourage her to talk through her feelings without invading her privacy.
- Validate her pain by reflecting back to the mother how you imagine she must feel.

  - "You must be heartbroken."
  - "I can't imagine the loss you feel."
  - "There is nothing more painful than what you are feeling right now."

- Try to key into the mother's needs and sense how often she would like to visit with you.
- Help her anticipate the stages of grief she will experience (see Figure 8-1).

Breastfeeding Concerns

- The mother may need comfort measures for engorgement.

  - Express enough milk for comfort without stimulating further milk production.
  - Continuous application of cabbage leaves will dry up the milk and offer relief; change the cabbage leaves every 2 to 3 hours.

- The mother may have been pumping or breastfeeding.

  - She may need to decrease pumping slowly in a weaning pattern.
  - She may wish to donate any expressed milk that was frozen.

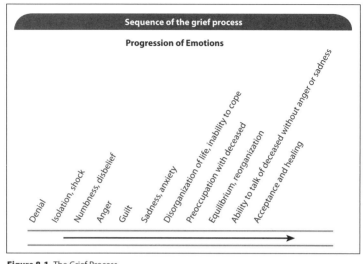

Figure 8-1 The Grief Process

Support for the Parents

- Emotional support:

  - Professional counseling through local clergy and social service organizations
  - Talking with other parents who have had similar experiences
  - Ongoing support from other parents and professionals in a support group

- Help them arrange time and privacy with their baby.
- Express your concern and sorrow.
- Use reflective listening and be available.
- Key into the mother's needs and sense how often she would like to hear from you.
- Help the mother relieve fullness without stimulating more milk production.
- Refer the mother to a milk bank if she wishes to donate her milk.
- Refer parents to a support system, and help them learn their rights and options.

ADVICE TO CLINICIANS

SUPPORT PARENTS

Parents' rights and options after a loss:

- ▶ Time and privacy with their baby
- ▶ The right to hold or see their baby after the loss
- ▶ Pictures of their baby for the parents to keep
- ▶ Baby's identification bracelet as a memento
- ▶ Baptism in the hospital
- ▶ Transportation arrangements to the funeral home

Box 8-1 COUNSELING GRIEVING PARENTS

DO show your genuine concern and caring.

DO be available to listen and empathize.

DO say you are sorry about what happened.

DO allow the mother to express as much grief as she feels.

DO encourage parents to be patient with themselves.

DO allow the mother to talk about her baby.

DO talk about the special qualities of the baby she lost.

DO acknowledge the impact of the baby's death.

DO reassure the parents that they did everything possible for their baby.

DO refer to the baby by name.

DO show your sadness and disappointment.

DON'T let your own sense of helplessness keep you from reaching out to the mother.

DON'T avoid the mother because you are uncomfortable with her situation.

DON'T say you know how the mother feels.

DON'T suggest that the mother should be feeling better by a certain time.

DON'T tell parents what they should feel or do.

DON'T change the subject when the baby is mentioned.

DON'T try to find something positive about the baby's death.

DON'T point out that they can always have other children or suggest that they should be grateful for any other children they already have.

DON'T suggest that the baby's care by the parents or medical personnel was inadequate.

DON'T avoid using the baby's name for fear of causing pain for the mother.

DON'T be overly cheerful or casual.

Source: Adapted with permission from a list compiled by the Compassionate Friends.

HIGH-RISK INFANTS

Tutorial for Students and Interns

Key Clinical Management Strategies

From *Clinical Guidelines for the Establishment of Exclusive Breastfeeding*, ILCA, 2005.

- Support exclusive breastfeeding during any illness or hospitalization of mother or infant.
- If medically indicated, provide additional nutrition using a method of supplementation that is least likely to compromise transition to exclusive breastfeeding.

Key Clinical Competencies

From *Clinical Competencies for IBCLC Practice* available at www.iblce.org.

- Assist mothers with preterm birth, including the benefits of kangaroo care.
- Assist mothers with traumatic birth.
- Assist mothers with infants born at 35–38 weeks gestation.
- Assist mothers with infants that are small or large for gestational age.
- Assist mothers who are coping with the death of an infant.

From Theory to Practice

1. Why might parents avoid contact with their high-risk infant?
2. How can you help parents increase interaction with their high-risk infant in the NICU?
3. Why are preterm infants at risk for jaundice?
4. How does skin-to-skin contact between a mother and baby facilitate breastfeeding?
5. What are the health benefits to a baby when held skin to skin with the mother?
6. Why is it important for preterm infants to receive their mother's milk?
7. What is the process for lactoengineering, and why is it used?
8. Why is freshly expressed milk preferred over frozen milk for a high-risk infant?
9. What pumping regimen would you recommend to the mother of a preterm infant?
10. What suggestions can you offer to a mother for increasing her milk production?
11. When can a preterm infant go to the breast?
12. Why is oxygen saturation better with breastfeeding than with bottle feeding?
13. What can a mother expect when her preterm infant first goes to the breast?
14. How can a mother help her baby's transition to feeding at the breast?
15. What help might a mother need from a lactation consultant when transitioning her preterm infant to the breast?
16. What are the parameters for discharging a preterm infant from the hospital?
17. What feeding plan would you develop for a mother who is taking her preterm infant home after a 3-week hospitalization?
18. A mother pumped her milk for 2 months while her preterm infant was hospitalized. Now that the baby is out of danger she tells you she plans to stop breastfeeding and feed the baby formula. How would you respond to her? What would be your first statement to her?
19. What are the risk factors for a late preterm infant relative to breastfeeding?
20. How can a mother ensure that her late preterm infant receives adequate nourishment?
21. How can the mother of a late preterm infant protect her milk production?
22. What role can a lactation consultant play in helping parents cope with the grief of losing their baby to a birth defect?

CHAPTER 9

Problem Solving

In This Chapter

Positioning and Latch Difficulty

Note: See Chapter 6 for signs of effective positioning and latch.

Improving Positioning

- Hold the baby in a position where the mother's dominant hand can bring the baby to breast quickly as soon as his or her mouth is opened wide.
- Hold the baby in a position where gravity can assist, such as the football hold.
- Use a prone position with chin support or sublingual pressure to avoid biting.
- Position the baby's head and shoulders in alignment facing the breast.
- Pull the baby's bottom closer to the mother's body to achieve better head flexion.
- Use a side-sitting position with the baby's head cradled in the mother's hand if the mother needs greater head control.

Helping with Latch

- Make sure the mother's breasts do not become so full they interfere with latch.
- Support the breast as needed to help the baby maintain a latch (see Figure 9-1).
- Flatten the breast to fit the plane of the baby's mouth (see Figure 9-2).
- Tickle the upper lip and slowly say "o...p...e...n" as the baby works to latch on.
- Drip milk onto the baby's lip or tongue.
- Place a finger with milk on it into the baby's mouth, pad side up.
- Attach the baby slightly off center so the baby takes in more of the underside of the nipple.
- Help the baby flange either or both lips when needed.
- Make sure the baby gets a deep latch with a mouthful of breast.

Everting a Flat or Inverted Nipple

- Wear breast shells between feedings to stretch the nipple forward.
- Form the nipple by hand or with the aid of ice just before a feeding.
- Stretch the nipple forward with a breast pump or other device before a feeding.
- Place a nipple shield over the nipple for the baby to pull the nipple forward. Then remove the shield and put the baby directly on the breast.

Encouraging the Baby to Feed

- Keep attempts to breastfeed very short and stop if the baby cries or pushes away.

  - Withdraw the breast, relax, reposition the baby and try again.
  - Try feeding on the other breast or holding the baby in a different position.
  - Snuggle skin to skin and watch for a return of approach behavior.

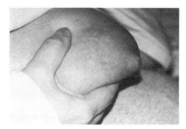

Figure 9-1 The C-Hold
Source: Printed with permission of Kay Hoover

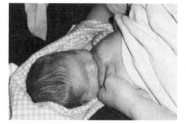

Figure 9-2 Compressing the Breast Like a Sandwich
Source: Printed with permission of Anna Swisher

- If the baby continually refuses to nurse:

    - Express milk to protect milk production.
    - Supplement with expressed milk with an alternative feeding method.
    - Use a nipple shield as a bridge to breastfeeding.

Disorganized Suckling

Select an Appropriate Intervention

- Begin with a course that places the baby in control.

    - If poor positioning is the cause, help the mother correct positioning.
    - Drip colostrum or glucose water onto the nipple to entice the baby.
    - Too much inappropriate intervention can result in oral aversion.

- Initiate techniques that are more intrusive only if they are necessary.

    - Insert an index finger in the baby's mouth to evaluate the oral cavity and suck.
    - Place an index finger in the baby's mouth to initiate rhythmic sucking.
    - Place light pressure on the midline of the tongue and pull the finger out slowly, verbally praising when the baby sucks it back in ("yes, that's right...").
    - Supplement with a feeding device at the breast to increase caloric intake and stimulate sucking.
    - Finger feed with a feeding tube.
    - Use a nipple shield as a bridge to direct breastfeeding.

- Make appropriate referrals.

    - Refer the baby for craniosacral therapy.
    - If ankyloglossia is present, help the mother find someone to clip the frenulum.
    - Refer to a specialist for suck training.

        ‣ The specialist places an index finger in the baby's mouth to stimulate portions of the oral anatomy to train the baby to suck.
        ‣ Suck training is not appropriate for an untrained clinician.
        ‣ Need for this intervention often occurs with other neurological problems.

Resolve the Cause

- Most feeding problems relate to poor latch and not to dysfunctional sucking.
- Consider potential consequences from treatment.

    - The baby can develop nipple preference from use of a bottle nipple.
    - Lower milk production can result from use of a nipple shield.
    - Feeding with special devices can become a chore for the mother.

PROBLEM SOLVING

Leaking
Causes of Leaking

- Overfull breasts
- Stimulation during lovemaking
- Overuse of breast shells
- Frequent milk expression
- Clothing that rubs against the nipples
- Overproduction of milk
- Hormone imbalance
- Psychological conditioning of letdown
- Hearing a baby cry
- Picking up the baby to nurse
- Thinking about breastfeeding or the baby
- Sexual orgasm

Controlling Leaking

- Use breast shells between feedings or on the opposite breast during a feeding.
- Press the heel of the hand over the breast or cross both arms and press.
- Wear absorbent breast pads and change them often.
- Feed the baby before lovemaking, and use absorbent towels over bedding.
- Decrease pressure from a bra by loosening it or wearing a larger size.
- Discontinue practices that stimulate the nipple.
- Express or pump milk when it is necessary to miss or delay a feeding.
- Wear dark, patterned clothing or a sweater to conceal moist spots.
- Discontinue medications or herbs that stimulate milk production.

Excessive or Inappropriate Leaking

- It may be a sign of an imbalance in other body functions.
- Milk production may greatly exceed the baby's needs.
- If after weaning or unrelated to birth or breastfeeding, it is galactorrhea (spontaneous lactation).
- Conditions that can cause galactorrhea:

  - Use of thyrotropin-releasing hormones, theophyllines, amphetamines, or tranquilizers
  - Chest or breast surgery
  - Fibrocystic breast
  - Herpes zoster
  - Breast stimulation
  - Sensitivity to normal levels of prolactin
  - An underlying health problem can elevate prolactin levels (hyperprolactinemia)

- Hypothyroidism
- Psychosis and anxiety medications
- Hyperthyroidism
- Chronic renal failure
- Pituitary tumors
- Uterine and ovarian tumors

Nipple Soreness

Transient Soreness or Nipple Pain

- Transient soreness occurs often with the initial latch and first few sucks.

  - Transient soreness peaks is between day 1 and day 6.
  - Hormonal changes occur postpartum.
  - The breast is adjusting to the frequency of use.

- Investigate all nipple pain.

  - Untreated nipple pain can progress to a crack.
  - Pain can decrease a woman's desire to put her baby to breast.

Causes of Nipple Pain

- Ineffective positioning and attachment are the main causes of nipple pain.
- Latch difficulty can cause soreness.

  - A near-term, SGA, LBW, or postmature infant with thin cheeks and little buccal fat pads has difficulty maintaining latch.
  - A tight frenulum (ankyloglossia) can prevent the tongue from extending over the lower lip (see Figure 9-3).
  - A tight labial frenum can interfere with flanging the upper lip (see Figure 9-4).
  - A short tongue may not extend far enough.

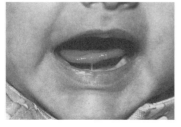

Figure 9-3 Tight Frenulum
Source: Printed with permission of Kay Hoover

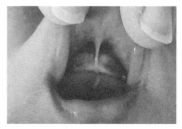

Figure 9-4 Tight Frenum
Source: Printed with permission of Anna Swisher

PROBLEM SOLVING

- The nipple can get caught in a high or bubble palate and not elongate far enough.
- Nipple shape or engorgement can make it difficult for the baby to latch.
- Use of an artificial bottle or pacifier nipple can cause poor latch.

- Improper use of a breast pump or nipple shield can damage the nipple.
- Pulling the baby off the breast without breaking suction can damage the nipple.
- An eager feeder with low milk flow can cause a "hicky" on the center of the mother's nipple.
- A strong letdown can cause the baby to clamp down or slide down onto the nipple.
- Nipple soreness can result from a skin condition such as thrush, impetigo, eczema, psoriasis, herpes, poison ivy, or a bacterial infection.
- Vasospasm of the nipple causes a Raynaud-like phenomenon that persists after the feeding, with stinging, tingling, burning pain, and triphasic color change (see Raynaud topic in Chapter 10).

Assessment of Nipple Soreness

- Obtain relevant information from the mother.

  - What is the baby's age, and is the baby teething?
  - When did the soreness begin?
  - How does the pain feel, and at what times does it hurt?

    - Burning pain may indicate thrush.
    - Throbbing may indicate mastitis.
    - Pain upon exposure to cold may indicate Raynaud's phenomenon.

  - What is the level of soreness?

    - Redness or bruising
    - Shallow crack or fissure, a compression stripe, or blister
    - Deep fissure or ulceration of the epidermis
    - Full erosion with damage throughout the dermis

  - Are there any chronic conditions or medication usage?
  - Has she changed soap, cream, lotion, laundry products, or perfume?

- Assess the breasts and nipples.

  - Are there signs of engorgement or infection (angry red streaks, swelling, pus)?
  - Is the nipple inverted or flat?
  - Does the nipple show signs of a poor latch after the baby has suckled for a few minutes?

    - The nipple is blanched and/or flattened.
    - The top of the nipple is rounded, and the bottom is flattened.

- Assess feeding technique.

    - Is the baby attached and positioned effectively?
    - Is the baby's body aligned and close to the breast?
    - Does the mother appear comfortable, with pillows for support?
    - Does the baby's mouth connect well with the breast?
    - Can the baby's tongue extend over the lower alveolar ridge?

Care Plan for Nipple Soreness

- Identify the cause, and correct mismanagement.

    - Respond to feeding cues promptly to avoid the baby being overly hungry.
    - Moisten the bra or breast pads before removing them if dried milk sticks to them.
    - Ensure effective positioning and a deep latch.
    - Form the nipple for the baby.
    - Break suction to reposition the baby if latch is ineffective.

- Provide palliative care.

    - Adjust feedings to reduce pain.

        ‣ Provide a lot of skin-to-skin contact.
        ‣ Initiate milk ejection before putting the baby to breast.
        ‣ Place ice in a wet cloth, and apply the cloth to the nipples prior to a feeding.
        ‣ Start a feeding with the least sore breast.
        ‣ Keep the baby's chin, and thus the tongue, away from the sore area.
        ‣ Use positions that will minimize further irritation (see Figure 9-5 for the most common positions and the resulting sore spots).

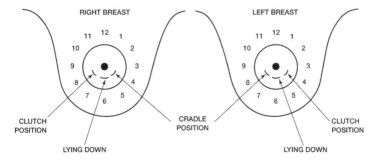

Figure 9-5 Location of Nipple Sore Related to Positioning

PROBLEM SOLVING

> ▸ Perform alternate massage to help sustain sucking and swallowing and relieve long periods of negative pressure.
> ▸ As the nipple improves, put the baby to breast for every second or third feeding and increase frequency as tolerated (see "Rest the nipple" below).
> ▸ Eliminate prolonged nonnutritive sucking.
> ▸ End the feeding when sucking slows, before the baby begins to chew on the nipple.

- Use a topical application on the nipple.

  > ▸ Apply colostrum or expressed milk after a feeding and air-dry.
  > ▸ Hypoallergenic medical grade anhydrous, or modified, lanolin may slow moisture loss and act as a moist wound healer.
  > ▸ Avoid topical agents that would further aggravate nipple damage.

    - High rates of infection may be associated with gel pads.
    - Regular lanolin contains pesticides.
    - Oils, including vitamin E, stay on the skin surface and do not facilitate moist wound healing.
    - Vitamin E in high doses can cause liver damage.

- Air-dry the nipples between feedings.
- Wear breast shells to promote healing.
- Consider an anti-inflammatory such as ibuprofen or acetaminophen.
- Treat a vasospasm.

  > ▸ Avoid cold and apply heat to the nipples after feeding.
  > ▸ Avoid caffeine and nicotine, which constrict blood vessels and increase the severity of vasospasm.
  > ▸ Increase intake of vitamin B_6 (no higher than 25 mg/day).
  > ▸ Consider a calcium channel blocker such as nifedipine.

- Rest the nipple.

  - Pump with an electric breast pump for several feedings to allow the nipple to heal.

    > ▸ Dab olive oil on the flange before pumping to lessen the pulling on the areola.
    > ▸ Begin pumping on the lowest suction and increase suction as the nipple improves.
    > ▸ Closely match feeding frequency.
    > ▸ Pump for 10 to 15 minutes every 2 to 3 hours.

  - Use a nipple shield for several feedings, pump to maintain milk production, and feed expressed milk to the baby by an alternative feeding method.

Cracked Nipples

- A crack or fissure can develop crosswise or lengthwise along the nipple.

  - A nipple that folds over causes a stress point at the fold.
  - Bleeding can occur when the baby stretches the nipple to the soft palate.
  - Blood from the nipple can cause the baby to vomit or have black stools.
  - An open wound is a pathway for bacteria.

- In addition to the treatment for sore nipples:

  - Cleanse the nipples.
  - Apply an antibacterial ointment such as mupirocin or polysporin.
  - Interrupt breastfeeding for 1 or 2 days until the nipples heal (see page 150, "Rest the nipple").
  - Culture the baby's throat and the mother's nipples for possible local infection.

Candidiasis

- *Candida albicans* is a fungal organism commonly found in the mouth, gastrointestinal tract, and vagina of healthy persons. The body's flora normally keeps the growth of *Candida* in check.
- The baby may contract a yeast infection during a vaginal delivery.

  - A yeast infection can cause the baby to seem gassy and fussy.
  - Yeast in the baby's mouth (thrush) presents as white patches that look like milk curds and cannot be wiped off.
  - Yeast in the diaper area can present as a raised, very red area with a sharply defined border.
  - Yeast in the vaginal area and vulva is tender and very red, with intense itching. It can produce a cheesy, white vaginal discharge.

- A yeast infection on the nipples is associated with:

  - Nipple damage early in lactation
  - Mastitis
  - Recent use of antibiotics in the postpartum period
  - Long-term antibiotic use before pregnancy
  - Vaginal yeast infection

- A yeast infection on the nipples does not always present with visual symptoms.

  - It is unusual to see white patches or redness on the nipple.
  - The most obvious symptom is intense, burning pain throughout the breast.
  - The areola may have a shiny, pinkish cast, detectable with a small flashlight.
  - The base of the nipple may have a break in the skin similar to a compression stripe.

- Treatment of a yeast infection:

  - Treat the baby's mouth, mother's nipples, and any other infection sites simultaneously.

    ‣ Rinse the baby's mouth with water after breastfeeding.

      – Shake and pour a topical agent into a cup.
      – Apply the agent to all surfaces of the baby's mouth with a cotton swab.

    ‣ Rinse the nipples with a solution of 1 cup of water and 1 tablespoon of vinegar.

      – Air-dry the nipples, and then apply the antifungal agent.
      – Expose the nipples to sunlight or artificial light briefly.
      – Change breast pads at every feeding.

  - Follow the full course of treatment even after symptoms subside.

    ‣ Over-the-counter agents:

      – Clotrimazole at 1%
      – Miconazole nitrate at 2%

> Conditions that can cause yeast infection:
> ‣ Diabetes
> ‣ Illness
> ‣ Pregnancy
> ‣ Oral contraceptive use
> ‣ Poor diet
> ‣ Antibiotic therapy
> ‣ Steroid therapy
> ‣ Immunosuppression
> ‣ Obesity
> ‣ Excessive sweating

Stopping the spread of yeast:

‣ Wash hands before and after diapering, after using the toilet, and after breastfeeding.
‣ Boil items that come in contact with the mother's breast, such as a bra, breast shells, or breast pump parts once a day for 20 minutes.
‣ Boil items that contact the baby's mouth, such as a pacifier, bottle nipple, or teething ring.
‣ Discard bottle nipples, pacifiers, and teethers after one week.
‣ Clean toys with hot soapy water.
‣ Launder the family's clothing in very hot water.
‣ Decrease dairy products and sugars in the mother's diet.
‣ Increase acidophilus, garlic, zinc, and B vitamins in the mother's diet.
‣ If the mother is sexually active, her partner may need treatment also.

‣ Prescription agents:

  – Nystatin
  – Ketoconazole at 2%
  – Ciclopirox at 1%
  – Naftifine hydrochloride

‣ Gentian violet is available from the pharmacist without a prescription.

  – Swab the baby's mouth with a 0.5% solution.
  – Put the baby to breast (thereby treating the nipple by contact).
  – Swab both breasts once daily.
  – Discontinue use after 7 days or earlier if pain subsides.

Engorgement
Normal Breast Fullness

- The breasts become fuller, heavier, and tender when milk production begins.
- Increased blood and lymph in the breast are sources of nutrients for milk production.
- Enlarged blood vessels are often visible beneath the skin.
- This fullness diminishes with unlimited, exclusive breastfeeding.
- The breasts become less full, soft, and pliable by about 10 days when lactation is established.

Overfullness in the Breast

- Symptoms of engorgement:

  ▪ The breasts are firm, hard, tender, and warm or hot to the touch.
  ▪ The skin is shiny and transparent.
  ▪ The nipples flatten and can be indistinguishable from the rest of the breast.

- Causes of engorgement:

  ▪ Failing to remove milk adequately or frequently enough
  ▪ Unnecessary regulations, schedules, and poor management of lactation
  ▪ Mother receiving IV fluids, creating edema in her feet and ankles as well
  ▪ Engorgement may occur any time during lactation

    ‣ The milk ducts do not clear of colostrum before mature milk begins.
    ‣ Breastfeeding is beginning and nursing patterns are irregular.
    ‣ The baby is sleeping through the night.
    ‣ The mother misses feedings because of separation from the baby.
    ‣ Weaning is occurring, especially if rapid weaning is necessary.

- Engorgement usually resolves within 12 to 24 hours with effective treatment.

PROBLEM SOLVING

Consequences of Engorgement

- The pressure on alveoli and milk ducts increases.

  - The flow of blood and lymph within the breast decreases.
  - Fewer nutrients become available to make milk.
  - The risk of infection increases because the breast does not remove bacteria at a normal rate.

- Engorgement can harm breast tissue permanently.

  - Alveolar cells and myoepithelial cells shrink and die off.
  - It can permanently compromise milk-producing ability for breastfeeding that baby.

- Production is inhibited by a suppressor peptide—feedback inhibitor of lactation (FIL).

  - Milk remaining in the breast for extended periods has a negative effect on milk production.
  - Milk secretion ceases during milk stasis and engorgement.

- Engorgement adversely affects letdown.

  - A flattened nipple becomes difficult for the baby to grasp.
  - The baby may not stimulate nerves in the nipple and areola sufficiently.
  - Without letdown, the baby cannot remove milk efficiently.

Preventing Engorgement

- Initiate breastfeeding within the first hour of life.
- Keep the mother and baby together 24 hours a day.
- Breastfeed in response to the baby's cues and for as long as the baby wants.
- Assess feeding practices for correct latch and positioning.
- Feed at least 10 to 12 times or more in 24 hours, including night feeds.
- Wake the baby and put him or her to breast to relieve fullness.
- Express milk after a feeding to remove remaining milk that flows quickly and easily.
- Avoid the use of artificial nipples.

Relieving Engorgement

- Compress the breast gently during feeds to encourage the baby to suckle.
- Express milk before the feeding to soften the areola.
- Relax in a warm shower, and hand express milk.
- Use reverse pressure softening to soften the areola and to enable the baby to latch.

Use of cabbage for relieving engorgement:

▶ Discard the outer leaves and pull off several inner leaves.

▶ Wash, pat dry, and crush the leaves slightly to break up the veins.

▶ Place the leaves around the breasts, leaving the nipple exposed.

▶ Hold the leaves in place with a bra.

▶ Refrigerate the remaining cabbage to keep it chilled for later use.

▶ Wear fresh leaves for 20 minutes every 2 hours, replacing wilted leaves as needed.

▶ Remove the cabbage when the breasts begin to feel tingly and cool, milk begins to leak, or the breast begins to soften.

▶ After removing the cabbage, put the baby to breast or pump if the baby still cannot latch.

▶ Discontinue cabbage when the baby or pumping provides needed relief.

▶ Some mothers use prolonged application of cabbage to wean.

• Apply cold compresses between feedings to help decrease discomfort.
• Have the mother lie flat on her back to elevate her breasts and help reduce swelling.
• Apply green cabbage leaves inside the bra.
• Express milk as needed between feedings, only removing milk that flows quickly and easily.

Pumping Guidelines for Engorgement

• Pumping is usually necessary for only 24 to 72 hours.
• Use a double electric pump, especially if the breasts feel hard and there is poor milk release.
• Pump before feeding if the areola is firm or hard, long enough to soften the areola for the baby.
• Pump after the feeding if needed.
• If milk removal is easy with audible gulping, pump until milk stops coming out quickly.
• If audible swallowing is sporadic, pump for 10 minutes and continue until milk flow slows.
• Apply cabbage or ice packs between feeding and pumping sessions to reduce swelling.
• Stop prefeed pumping as soon as possible, and pump after feeding only when necessary.

PROBLEM SOLVING

Plugged Duct

What Is a Plug?

- A plug contains cells and other milk components shed within the duct.
- It causes localized soreness, swelling, lumpiness, or slight pain.
- The plug may be absorbed and not appear in the milk.
- The plug may come out as brownish, greenish, thick and stringy.
- The baby may reject the breast with the plug due to taste or texture of the milk.
- If not treated quickly, a plug could develop into a caked breast or mastitis.

> Avoiding a recurrence of plugged ducts:
>
> ▶ Reduce saturated fats in the mother's diet.
> ▶ Add lecithin to the mother's diet:
>   - 1 tablespoon three or four times a day
>   - 1 to 2 capsules (1200 milligrams each) three or four times a day

Causes of a Plugged Duct

- A plug results from incomplete milk removal or a practice that inhibits free flow of milk.
- Practices that place outside pressure on specific areas of the breast:

    - A tight or underwire bra, bunched up clothing under the arm, or a baby sling.
    - Consistently feeding, holding, carrying, or rocking the baby in the same position.
    - Sleeping in a position that puts pressure on the breast.
    - Repeated pressure from a breast pump flange.

Treatment of a Plugged Duct

- Establish regular, frequent feedings.
- Begin a feeding on the breast with the plug for the more vigorous sucking.
- Use a position where the baby's tongue stimulates the area of the plug.
- Massage from the plug toward the nipple.
- Place moist heat over the area of the plug.

Milk Blister

What Is a Milk Blister?

- A clog of milk in a nipple pore prevents milk from flowing from that duct.
- A milk blister is intensely painful.
- It is a milk bleb or blocked nipple pore when it is open.
- It is a nipple blister or milk blister when skin closes over the pore.

Removing a Blister

- Soak the nipple with a warm, wet compress or in a warm bowl of water.
- Gently rub it with a washcloth to remove the pore covering; nurse the baby to remove the plug.
- Open it with a sterile needle immediately after a feed; compress the breast to aid in drainage.
- Apply a topical antibiotic ointment to avoid infection.
- Breastfeed frequently and thoroughly to prevent recurrence.
- Milk stasis with a blister can lead to mastitis.

Mastitis

What Is Mastitis?

- Mastitis is inflammation of the breast, usually from a bacterial infection.
- The most frequent site is the upper, outer quadrant unilaterally.
- The infection is usually located outside the ducts in surrounding breast tissue.
- The inflamed area becomes red, hot, and tender to the touch.
- Mastitis usually produces a fever and flulike symptoms.
- The baby may reject the infected breast.

Causes of Mastitis

- The mother's immunity is lower because of pregnancy; she feels fatigue or stress.
- An interruption in breastfeeding or change in pattern causes milk to remain in the breast.
- A crack in the nipple provides a pathway for *Staphylococcus* and other organisms.
- Milk stasis, engorgement, an untreated plugged duct, or trauma leads to an infection.
- Bacteria in the baby's mouth or the home environment lead to an infection.

Treatment of Mastitis

- Adjust breastfeeding management.

  - Apply warm, moist compresses to the inflamed area before and during feedings.
  - Begin feedings on the affected breast for more vigorous sucking.
  - Point the baby's chin toward the inflamed area.
  - Drain the breast by feeding frequently and as long as the baby wants.
  - Massage and compress the breast to help with drainage.
  - Express remaining milk from the affected breast after every feeding.

- Treat the infection and pain.

- Take anti-inflammatory medication for comfort.
- Obtain an antibiotic if the infection does not resolve in 24 hours and the mother has a temperature higher than 100°F (37°C).
- Get bed rest, and request time off work if the mother works.
- Soak the breast in warm water for short periods to facilitate blood flow and milk drainage.

- If the infection does not resolve or recurs:

  - Obtain a stronger or broader-spectrum antibiotic.
  - Culture the milk, the nipple, and the baby's throat to determine an appropriate antibiotic.

Causes of recurrent mastitis:

▶ Bacteria may be resistant to the antibiotic.

▶ The mother does not follow the entire course of treatment.

▶ Anemia or other deficiencies predispose some women to recurrent mastitis.

▶ The mother needs to improve her hygiene, diet, rest, or exercise.

▶ The mother is overly committed or stressed.

▶ The mother lacks support among family or friends.

Abscessed Breast

- What is an abscessed breast?

  - An abscess is a localized collection of pus.
  - The infection site becomes red, swollen, and tender.
  - It causes fever, flulike symptoms, nausea, extreme fatigue, and aching muscles.
  - Symptoms are less severe than with mastitis because the abscess is isolated.
  - An abscess can occur in the absence of systemic symptoms.
  - An abscess can be a serious health hazard that requires physician referral for treatment.

- Treatment is usually to lance and drain the abscess and prescribe medication for the infection.
- Continued breastfeeding depends on the location of the abscess, pain level, and medication.

  - The mother can pump the affected breast until the abscess heals. A breast pump manufacturer can modify a flange so it does not rub on the abscess.
  - The mother can wean on the affected breast and continue with one-sided nursing.

Insufficient Milk Production

Perceived Insufficiency

- Milk production is the most common concern for mothers.
- The mother may be unfamiliar with newborn behavior.

  - The baby nurses frequently.
  - The baby does not seem satisfied and is fussy after feedings.

- The mother lacks confidence:

  - In her ability to provide sufficient nourishment
  - In her competence as a parent
  - That her milk is rich enough or satisfying enough
  - That her milk might be causing an allergic response or excessive gas

Signs of Sufficient Milk Production

- By day 4, the baby has at least six wet and three soiled diapers in each 24-hour period.

  - Urine is pale and dilute.
  - Stools are yellow or turning yellow.
  - This pattern continues until 5 to 6 weeks of age.

- The baby routinely nurses at least eight times in each 24-hour period.

  - The breasts feel softer after a feeding.
  - The nipples are not painful during or after feedings.
  - The baby's sucking rhythm slows as milk flows.
  - The mother hears swallowing or gulping.

- The baby's weight and disposition:

  - The baby regains birth weight by 10 to 14 days.
  - The baby gains 4 to 8 ounces a week.
  - The baby is alert and active, and is content between feedings.
  - The baby usually rests for 1 to 2 hours, and then wakes to nurse again.

Increasing Milk Production

- Most insufficient milk results from ineffective breastfeeding.
- Factors in a mother's ability to increase milk production:

  - Age of the baby
  - Willingness of the baby to nurse
  - Degree of breast involution

- Condition of the baby
- The amount of any supplements the baby is receiving
- The mother's motivation to increase frequency of feedings

- Measures to increase milk production:

  - Keep the baby skin to skin as much as possible for 48 hours.
  - Nurse lying down, and rest between feedings.
  - Alternate between breasts several times during a feeding.
  - Resume night feedings if they were dropped.
  - Pump milk with an electric breast pump between feedings.
  - Increase protein, fresh fruits, vegetables and B vitamins in the mother's diet.
  - Use a galactagogue such as fenugreek, blessed thistle, domperidone, or metoclopramide.

Concerns About Infant Growth
Normal Patterns in a Healthy Infant

- Birth weight doubles by 4 months and triples by 12 months.
- Body length increases by 50% at 12 months.
- Head circumference increases by 7.6 cm (3 inches) at 1 year.
- The baby has frequent voids and stools in the first month and less frequent thereafter.
- The baby has bright eyes, an alert manner, and good muscle and skin tone.

Signs of Inadequate Growth

- Weight:

  - Weight loss continues after the third day for a full-term infant.
  - There is no weight gain by day 4.
  - Weight loss is beyond 10–15% in the first week (see Appendix H).
  - The baby is not back to birth weight by 10 to 14 days.

- Output:

  - The baby is still passing meconium after day 4.
  - A baby under 5 to 6 weeks of age passes few stools.
  - Urine is decreased or concentrated.
  - Urine in an older baby smells strongly of ammonia.

- The baby's disposition:

  - The baby sleeps for long periods to conserve energy.
  - The baby fusses when removed from the breast and falls asleep when put back to breast.

- The baby cannot be put down without fussing.
- The baby nurses infrequently or constantly.
- The baby has few periods of quiet, alert time.
- The baby has a worried or anxious facial appearance.
- The baby stays in a flexed fetal position to maintain temperature.
- The baby has hanging folds of skin on the thighs and buttocks.
- The baby has a high-pitched cry that sounds like the "mew" of a cat.

Newborn Dehydration

- A newborn who does not receive enough fluids can become dehydrated.

  - Follow up with mothers and babies who go home early.
  - Evaluate breastfeeding technique.
  - Document the baby's feedings, stools, and voids.
  - Weigh the baby before and after feedings on a digital electronic scale to assess milk transfer.

- Symptoms of dehydration:

  - Few or no stools
  - Scant urinary output
  - The baby sleeps at the breast
  - Infrequent feedings
  - Weight loss greater than 10–15% of birth weight
  - Lethargy
  - A weak cry
  - Dry mucous membranes
  - No tears
  - Poor skin turgor
  - Sunken fontanels

Slow Weight Gain

- Intervention is unnecessary with a healthy pattern.

  - Growth is slow and steady over time.
  - Growth is proportional for weight, length, and head circumference.
  - The baby's development is age appropriate.

- Determine the need for intervention.

  - Evaluate the mother's breastfeeding technique.
  - Review feeding behavior and investigate the baby's feeding pattern.
  - Confirm that feeds are unrestricted and the baby receives no pacifiers or bottles.
  - Record the baby's weights to monitor growth.

PROBLEM SOLVING

Poor Weight Gain

- Indication of poor weight gain:

  - The newborn remains below birth weight by several ounces at day 14.
  - An older baby is not gaining or is gaining less than 3 ounces per week.

- Pre- and postweights can determine ineffective milk removal or low milk production.

  - If milk production is low:

    - Supplemental tube feeding accomplishes two goals simultaneously.

      - Supplements the baby with donor milk or formula
      - Increases the level of milk production to a level that sustains the baby

    - Pump immediately after feeds.
    - Slowly decrease the amount of supplement as the baby gains weight.

  - If milk production is sufficient and milk removal is ineffective, pump after feedings and feed the milk to the baby to increase calories and improve feeding efficiency.

- Counseling and documentation:

  - Approach mothers with sensitivity, validation, and reassurance.
  - If parents supplement with a bottle, teach them paced feeding to slow flow rate.
  - Caution against the use of pacifiers so sucking is at the breast.
  - Record the baby's weight at least twice a week to monitor gain.
  - Send a report of the feeding plan to the baby's and mother's caregivers.

Failure to Thrive (FTT)

- Signs:

  - The baby continues to lose weight after day 10.
  - The baby does not regain birth weight by week 3.
  - Weight gain is below the 10th percentile after 1 month.
  - Growth deviates downward by 2 major percentiles on the growth chart.
  - The baby is lethargic, hypertonic, irritable and difficult to soothe, sleeps excessively, or is continuously fussy.

- Causes:

  - Breastfeeding management or technique is ineffective.
  - The baby is sleepy or placid and does not display appropriate feeding behavior.
  - The baby is preterm, SGA, or has neuromotor problems.
  - The baby has a tight frenulum or disorganized suck.

- The mother's breast anatomy and the infant's oral anatomy connect ineffectively.
- The mother has a condition or had surgery that disrupted milk flow or nerve pathways.
- The mother has PCOS, hypoprolactinemia, Sheehan's syndrome, retained placental fragments, or a hormonal disorder.

- Assessment:

  - Assess the baby's latch, sucking technique, and position at the breast.
  - Assess the baby's mouth for an oral anomaly such as ankyloglossia.
  - Assess milk transfer with pre- and postfeed weights.
  - See Figure 9-6 for questions to ask to assess failure to thrive.

- Interventions may be required for a long time.

  - Watch for and respond to signs of hunger.
  - Nurse 10–12 times in 24 hours around the clock until the baby has three stools per 24 hours for 3 days in a row.
  - Switch breasts when the baby's suckling pattern changes and swallowing ceases.
  - Compress the breast to increase milk flow during feeds.
  - Limit feeds to 40 minutes per session.
  - Supplement after every feed until the baby is gaining well, per caregiver guidelines.
  - Pump with a double electric pump for 15 minutes immediately after.
  - Nurse at least once during the night to take advantage of higher prolactin levels.
  - Ensure that the baby visits the caregiver frequently.
  - Record the baby's weight frequently.
  - Communicate closely with the lactation consultant and the baby's caregiver.

- Supplementation:

  - Determine total daily requirements and divide into the number of feedings (see Table 9-1).
  - Obtain pre- and postfeed weights to determine the amount of supplement needed.

    - Weigh the baby 2 hours after the previous feeding and milk expression.
    - Weigh the baby after the feeding and record the amount of milk consumed.
    - Pump both breasts, record the amount of residual milk, and feed it to the baby.
    - Subtract the amount of milk consumed from the requirement for that feeding to determine the amount of supplement needed.

  - Pump after a feed to collect residual milk, feed it to the baby, and supplement as necessary with expressed milk or formula.

Questions to ask for assessing failure to thrive	
Ask:	**For the possibility of:**
How much weight did you gain during pregnancy?	Low fat in the mother's milk or an eating disorder
How did your breasts change during pregnancy?	Sufficient mammary tissue
Do you have a history of infertility or miscarriages?	Thyroid disorder
Are you aware of having any thyroid dysfunction?	Thyroid disorder
Have you had any breast procedure, such as a biopsy, cyst removal, augmentation, or reduction? Have you ever had a breast injury?	Severed milk ducts
Were there any complications during delivery?	Excessive blood loss or the use of Pitocin or IV fluids
Are you using oral contraceptives?	Low milk production
What did you eat yesterday?	Poor dietary intake
Do you smoke cigarettes? How many per day?	Low milk production
How much alcohol do you drink and how often?	Low milk production
Have you experienced any breast engorgement or mastitis?	Previous milk stasis that lowered prolactin receptor sites
Describe your breastfeeding routine.	Insufficient feeding frequency or duration
How much does your baby use a pacifier?	Reduced breastfeeding
How much time does your baby spend in a swing?	Reduced breastfeeding
Is there a particular parenting program or schedule that you are trying to follow?	Restrictive baby training program

Figure 9-6 Questions to Ask for Assessing Failure to Thrive

Table 9-1 Determining the Number of Ounces an Infant Needs

Example for an infant weighing 4 pounds and 2 ounces	
Convert infant's weight to ounces.	4 lb + 2 oz = 66 oz
Divide total ounces by 6 to determine amount required for 24-hour intake.	66 oz ÷ 6 = 11 oz
Divide the 24-hour requirements by the number of feedings per 24-hour period to determine how much is required per feeding.	11 oz ÷ 8 feedings = 1.37 oz per feeding 11 oz ÷ 6 feedings = 1.83 oz per feeding

- Reduce supplements slowly and continue with an increased number of breastfeeds.

  - Record the amount of supplement, number of breastfeeds, and wet and soiled diapers.
  - Decrease the amount of supplement slowly, with frequent weight checks.
  - Never dilute formula to cut back on supplements.
  - Discontinuing supplements can take several weeks of concentrated effort.

Tutorial for Students and Interns

Key Clinical Management Strategies

From *Clinical Guidelines for the Establishment of Exclusive Breastfeeding*, ILCA, 2005.

- If medically indicated, provide additional nutrition using a method of supplementation that is least likely to compromise transition to exclusive breastfeeding.
- Identify maternal and infant risk factors that may affect the mother's or infant's ability to breastfeed effectively and provide appropriate assistance and follow-up.

Key Clinical Competencies

From *Clinical Competencies for IBCLC Practice* available at www.iblce.org.

- Identify situations in which immediate verbal communication with the healthcare provider is necessary, such as serious illness in the infant, child, or mother.
- Identify the mother's concerns or problems, planned interventions, evaluation of outcomes and follow-up.

PROBLEM SOLVING

- Instruct the mother about prevention and treatment of engorgement.
- Instruct the mother about prevention and treatment of sore nipples.
- Assess and evaluate the infant's ability to breastfeed.
- Assess effective milk transfer.
- Evaluate effectiveness of the breastfeeding plan.
- Assess contributing factors and etiology of problems.
- Develop an appropriate breastfeeding plan in concert with the mother, and assist the mother to implement the plan.
- Assist mothers with maintaining and increasing milk production.
- Assist mothers with yeast infections of the breast, nipple, areola, and milk ducts.
- Assist mothers with nipple pain and damage.
- Assist mothers with engorgement.
- Assist mothers with a plugged duct or blocked nipple pore.
- Assist mothers with mastitis.
- Assist mothers with insufficient milk supply, differentiating between perceived and real.
- Assist mothers with an infant at high risk for hypoglycemia.
- Assist mothers with excessive weight loss, slow or poor weight gain.
- Assist mothers with yeast infection.
- Assist mothers with an infant with tonic bite or ineffective or dysfunctional suck.
- Assist mothers with flat or inverted nipples.
- Demonstrate appropriate use and understanding of potential disadvantages or risks of use of:

  - Herbal supplements for mother or infant
  - Nipple creams and ointments
  - Breast shells
  - Breast pumps
  - Alternative feeding techniques
  - Tube feeding at the breast
  - Cup feeding
  - Spoon feeding
  - Eyedropper feeding
  - Finger feeding
  - Nipple shields
  - Infant scales
  - A device to evert nipples

From Theory to Practice
Feeding Problems

1. How can you help a mother protect her milk production when her baby has trouble latching on?

2. What measures would you take to help a mother whose nipples are too flat for the baby to achieve a latch?
3. Remembering that you need to limit the amount of suggestions at one time, what would your initial plan be for a mother whose baby is still having difficulty maintaining a latch at day 2? What would be your first statement to her?
4. The mother of a 36-hour-old infant is in tears because she continually struggles getting her baby latched on for feeds. The nurses have tried to help, and this is the first time a lactation consultant has seen her. How will you help her? What will be your first statement to her?
5. Why is skin-to-skin care helpful for a baby who has difficulty latching on for feeds?
6. You observe a 24-hour-old infant who has a good latch but sucks on his or her tongue during feeds. How will you help the mother?
7. What is the procedure for assessing an infant's suck?
8. When is it appropriate to assess an infant's suck digitally? What would you look for?
9. What is the appropriate use of a nipple shield for a baby who has difficulty achieving a good latch?

Nipple Problems

1. How would you help a mother who tells you it is always painful when she takes the baby off her nipple? What would be your first statement to her?
2. How does transient nipple soreness differ from positional soreness?
3. You take breast pads to a mother on the third day postpartum and she complains that her nipples just started to get sore. You observe a feed and confirm that her baby has good positioning and latch. What else will you explore and what suggestions will you offer her?
4. You observe a feed and note that the mother's nipple appears blanched when her baby releases the nipple. She complains that it is tender. What do you suspect is happening, and what do you suggest to the mother?
5. You have been asked to update the hospital protocol for nipple soreness. What treatment regimen will you recommend and in what order?
6. You see a mother at 2 weeks postpartum for severely cracked nipples. What will you investigate, and what palliative care will you recommend?
7. What will you investigate in trying to determine if yeast is the cause of a mother's sore nipples?
8. How would you expect the rate of thrush infections of babies born by cesarean to compare with that of babies who are born vaginally?
9. A mother complains of a stinging pain on her nipples after feedings. You examine her nipples and do not see any signs of a yeast infection. Her baby shows no signs of thrush. What might be the cause of her nipple pain?

10. You determine that a mother has a yeast infection on her nipple and recommend treatment for both her nipples and her baby's mouth. Why would you treat a baby's mouth for thrush if there is no sign of infection?
11. What dietary adjustments can a mother make when she has a yeast infection on her nipples?

Breast Problems

1. Juliette and her infant, Matthew, were discharged at 48 hours postpartum. Her nipples were slightly tender at discharge. You call 3 days later to follow up. She tells you that her nipples feel better, but now she is having a problem with her breasts leaking. What will you investigate?
2. Juliette returns to work when Matthew is 2 months old. Her breasts leak continually when she is at work. What will you investigate, and what suggestions will you offer her?
3. A mother's breasts become more full at around 3–4 days postpartum, as milk production begins. Why does this initial fullness subside by about 10 days?
4. How does the initial fullness with the onset of milk production differ from breast engorgement?
5. A baby has difficulty latching on for feeding when milk production causes the mother's breasts to become full and rounded. What plan of care will you recommend?
6. How does milk expression before and after a feeding help with engorgement?
7. What precautions would you give to mothers about protecting their milk production when using cabbage?
8. What are the possible consequences of severe breast engorgement?
9. What can you teach mothers at discharge to help them avoid engorgement after they go home?
10. Jennifer had problems with breast engorgement at 4 days when milk production began. You follow up at 1 week postpartum and learn that her breasts are not as full between feedings. She mentions that when she massages her left breast she feels a small bump near her underarm. She asks if it is a normal part of breastfeeding. What is your response and plan of care?
11. Jennifer also asks why she would develop a pimple on the end of her nipple. What is your response and plan of care?
12. What is the relationship between breast engorgement and mastitis?
13. You have determined that Heather has mastitis. She is worried about the safety of continuing to breastfeed her baby because of the infection. What is your response and plan of care?
14. Heather calls you with her third case of mastitis and wonders what she can do to stop getting a breast infection. What is your response, and what will you investigate?

15. What is the relationship between mastitis and a breast abscess, and how do the symptoms differ?
16. How do feeding recommendations differ between mastitis and a breast abscess?

Problems with Milk Production and Infant Growth

1. How can you ensure that mothers in your care do not worry needlessly about sufficient milk production?
2. A mother's baby has been too sleepy to breastfeed ever since birth 3 days ago. What measures can you take to ensure that the mother establishes and maintains full milk production?
3. Genevieve's baby, Cole, weighed 7 lb 12 oz at birth. At 1 month, Cole weighs 8 lb 4 oz. Genevieve asks if she should worry about her milk production. What is your response and what will you investigate?
4. Janet's baby, Lucas, is 2 ounces shy of regaining his birth weight at 2 weeks. Is there a concern, and what feeding recommendations would you make, if any?
5. You determine that a mother of a 3-week-old infant has inadequate milk production. What do you need to investigate before you can recommend a plan of care?
6. Sandra's baby is still passing meconium at day 4. What do you need to investigate?
7. Ann Marie brings her 1-month-old son Rob to see you. Rob has been exclusively breastfed since birth. Ann Marie is concerned that he continually falls asleep at the breast. Rob weighed 8 lb 5 oz at birth. When you weigh him, his weight is 8 lb 5 oz. What will you investigate, and what feeding recommendations will you make?
8. What parameters determine that a baby is a slow gainer rather than having poor weight gain?
9. Susan was told to respond to her baby's feeding behavior. She has fed him whenever he demonstrated feeding behavior. When you weigh him, you learn that he has not regained his birth weight at 3 weeks. What could be the cause, and what would you recommend to Susan?
10. How will you determine that supplements are no longer needed for a baby who is failing to thrive?

CHAPTER 10

Techniques and Devices

In This Chapter

Techniques Used for Breastfeeding

Nipple Compression

- Purpose: Assess nipples for ability to extend outward. A normal nipple moves forward. An inverted nipple moves inward.
- Method: Grasp the base of the nipple with the forefinger and thumb and press together.

Breast Massage

- Purpose: Help the mother relax, become familiar with the normal lumps of a lactating breast, and stimulate milk flow and letdown.
- Method: Exert gentle pressure with the palm of the hand in a circular motion from the chest wall toward the nipple. Work the hand around the breast, focusing under the breast and along the side under the arm—the areas of greatest milk duct development.

Breast Compression

- Purpose: Push milk down the ducts during a feed to encourage sustained sucking.
- Method: Hold the breast with the thumb on top and the fingers cupping the bottom. When the baby is no longer sucking nutritively, squeeze the breast gently to trigger another sucking burst.

Reverse Pressure Softening (See Table 10-1)

Table 10-1 Reverse Pressure Softening Technique

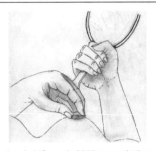

One handed "flower hold." Fingernails short, fingertips curved, placed where the baby's tongue will go.

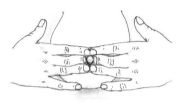

Two handed, one-step method. Fingernails short, fingertips curved, each one touching the side of nipple.

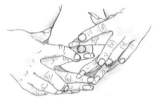

The mother may ask someone to help press by placing fingers or thumbs on top of hers.

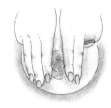

Two step method, two hands, using 2 or 3 straight fingers on each side, first knuckles touching the nipple. Move ¼ turn, repeat above and below the nipple.

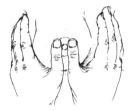

Two step method, two hands, using straight thumbs, base of the thumbnail even with the side of the nipple. Move ¼ turn, repeat, thumbs above and below the nipple.

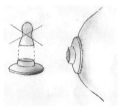

Soft ring method. Cut off the bottom half of an artificial nipple to place on the areola to press with fingers.

Source: Printed by permission of Lactation Education Consultants, © 2004. May be reproduced for non-commercial purposes. Illustrations by Kyle Cotterman

Breast Sandwich

- Purpose: Support and shape the breast for feedings and keep the nipple from slipping out of the baby's mouth.
- Method: Place the thumb opposite the fingers well behind the areola so the fingers do not interfere with latch. Compress the breast to make a "sandwich" in line with the baby's mouth.

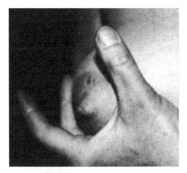

Dancer Hand Position
(See Figure 10-1)

- Purpose: For babies with weak muscle development, to hold the jaw steady while they suck
- Method: Support the baby's chin in the crook of the hand between the thumb and index finger. Gently hold the baby's cheeks to increase negative pressure, and support the underside of the breast with the other three fingers. As muscle tone improves, move the thumb to the top of the breast and support the baby's chin with the index finger.

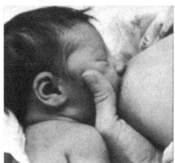

Figure 10-1 Dancer Hand Position
Source: Printed with permission of Sarah Coulter Danner

Manual Expression
(See Figure 10-2)

- Purpose: Remove colostrum or milk from the breast to lubricate skin or to collect milk.
- Method:
  - Wash your hands and gently massage the breast. Apply a warm, moist cloth for several minutes to promote milk flow.
  - Lean slightly forward with the nipple aimed at the collection container.

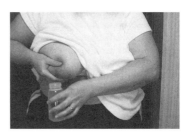

Figure 10-2 Mother Removing Her Milk by Hand Expression
Source: Printed with permission of Anna Swisher

TECHNIQUES AND DEVICES

- Place the thumb and index finger opposite each other about 1½ inch from the tip of the nipple. Press the thumb and index finger back toward the chest wall. Gently press the thumb and finger together and pull forward.
- As milk flow subsides, massage the breast again, reposition the thumb and finger around the breast and repeat.

Devices Used for Breastfeeding

Lubricant

- Purpose: Heal sore nipples.
- Method: Massage a small amount of colostrum, breastmilk, or hypoallergenic medical grade anhydrous lanolin into the nipple and areola after a feeding. Air-dry for 10 minutes. The lubricant will be absorbed before the next feeding.
- Considerations: Avoid substances that inhibit skin respiration or are drying such as vitamin E, petroleum, or alcohol. Avoid potential allergens such as peanut oil, massé cream, or wool derivatives.

Inverted Syringe for Flat or Inverted Nipple (See Figure 10-3)

- Purpose: Help evert a flat or inverted nipple
- Method:

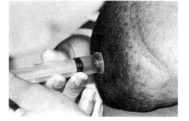

Figure 10-3 Inverted Syringe Used to Pull Out the Nipple
Source: Printed with permission of Kay Hoover

  - Select a syringe with a barrel slightly larger than the nipple (10–20 ml).
  - Cut off the tapered end of the syringe and reverse the plunger direction so the smooth surface is against the breast.
  - Pull gently on the plunger to help the nipple protrude before putting the baby to breast.
  - Wash the syringe in hot, soapy water after the feeding and air-dry for the next use.

Breast Shells

- Purpose: Help shape a flat or inverted nipple and protect and air-dry sore nipples.

- Method: Place the shells over the nipples inside the bra with the openings on top. Avoid excessive use or wearing shells while sleeping.

Nipple Shield

- Purpose: Assist with latching or suckling difficulties.
- Method:

  - Fold the shield back so it is almost inside out and place it snugly over the nipple with the nipple centered in the shield. Keep the shield in place briefly at the beginning of the feed, remove it after the baby begins to suckle, and then quickly put the baby directly on the breast. Attempt to put the baby directly to breast periodically, with a goal to discontinue the shield.

- Considerations:

  - Try other techniques first: change positioning, form the nipple, reduce breast fullness, or use eversion techniques.
  - Use of a shield can help with the following:

    - Compensating for lack of fat buccal pads and weak suckle
    - Forming flat or inverted nipples that do not respond to other attempts to improve latch
    - The transition to direct breastfeeding when a baby refuses the breast

  - Use an appropriate shield.

    - Select the smallest size that accommodates the baby's mouth and the mother's nipple.
    - Use only silicon material.
    - Never try to force a large, prominent nipple into a small shield.

  - A preterm or low-birth-weight infant may need the shield in place for the entire feeding to transfer milk.
  - Precautions when using a nipple shield:

    - Obtain help from a lactation consultant.
    - Check the baby's weight periodically.
    - Pump to maintain milk production.
    - Monitor the baby's intake and output.

Breast Pump

- Purpose: Relieve breast fullness, collect milk, and increase milk production.
- Handheld breast pump:

- Use for short-term or occasional removal of milk, or to shape the nipple before feeding.
- The pump includes a collecting bottle and flange that fits over the breast.
- A piston, trigger, or motor provides suction.
- It comes as a manual pump, battery-operated pump, or a combination of battery and electric.

- Electric breast pump:

  - Use for regular absence of nursing when the mother and baby cannot be together, or to shape the nipple before feeding.
  - This pump most closely mimics the baby's suckling rhythm and nipple stimulation.
  - A double pump reduces pumping time and increases breast stimulation.
  - The mother either purchases a personal pump kit and rents a pump, or purchases a pump, which includes all parts.

- Pumping technique:

  - Wash hands, get comfortable, and massage the breasts briefly.
  - Express a few drops of milk to help milk letdown and encourage faster results.
  - Select a flange size or use an insert to accommodate breast size and allow the nipple to move freely.
  - Moisten the pump flange with milk or olive oil to provide a better seal.
  - Center the nipple in the flange and ensure that breast tissue touches the sides.
  - If using an electric pump, begin with suction on the lowest setting and increase suction strength according to comfort.

- Pumping time:

  - Prolactin levels are highest during sleep. Pumping when she wakes during the night or in early morning may yield more milk than pumping in the afternoon or evening.
  - Pumping may be in place of a missed feeding, between feedings, or on one breast while feeding on the other breast.
  - When the baby is unable to nurse, pump eight times every 24 hours to maintain and protect milk production.

    - If double pumping, pump for 12–15 minutes.
    - If single pumping, alternate breasts several times to total 12–15 minutes.

- Encouraging milk to release:

  - Pump when rested and unhurried.
  - Arrange for privacy and a comfortable chair.
  - Listen to relaxing music.
  - Have a picture of the baby and a tape recording of the baby's sounds.

Criteria for selecting a breast pump:

▶ Does it cycle quickly, similar to the rhythm of an infant's suck?

▶ Is the flange shape comfortable and an appropriate size for the mother's breast?

▶ Are larger and smaller flanges or inserts available?

▶ Will the pump accommodate standard bottles for collecting milk?

▶ Are the parts dishwasher-safe?

▶ Is the pump easy to assemble?

▶ Is the pump easy and comfortable to use?

▶ If the pump is electric, will the power source be adequate?

▶ Is the pump quiet?

▶ Is the pump easy to transport?

▶ Is the pump affordable for the length of time it is required?

▶ Are quick service and overnight replacement available?

▶ What period and what parts does the warranty cover?

▶ Are written instructions provided?

▶ Is there someone knowledgeable in breastfeeding to answer questions and resolve problems?

▶ Is there an up-to-date Web site?

- Avoid watching the pump or breast while pumping.
- Ensure that the nipple has contact with the side of the flange.

Pacifier

- Purpose:

  - Provide sucking for a preterm infant during gavage feeding.
  - Calm an infant who must undergo a painful procedure.
  - Comfort an infant with gastroesophageal reflux disease (GERD).

- Considerations:

  - Inadequate time spent at the breast can reduce milk production, cause poor weight gain, or cause insufficient breast drainage resulting in engorgement or mastitis.
  - Sucking on a pacifier can tire the baby or increase hunger to the point of crying.
  - Pacifier use can cause parents to miss feeding behavior.
  - Pacifier use should not replace feeding or interaction and skin contact.

- Alternatives:

  - Respond to early feeding behavior to prevent crying.
  - Insert the index finger, pad side up, very gently into the baby's mouth and allow the baby to draw the finger in to the first knuckle (see Figure 10-4).
  - Use a baby sling or other comfort aid.

Alternate Feeding Methods

Spoon Feeding (See Figure 10-5)

- Considerations: Useful for rousing a baby for early feedings and for collecting milk when teaching hand expression.
- Method: Express colostrum into a spoon. Lay the tip of the spoon gently at the tip of the baby's tongue. Ladle colostrum onto the baby's tongue a few drops at a time.

Tube Feeding at the Breast

- Considerations:

  - The least invasive supplemental feeding method.
  - The baby is encouraged to suckle by the flow of milk at the breast.
  - The mother receives breast stimulation to encourage milk production.
  - Noncommercial supplementer: A number 5, 6, or 8 French oral gastric tube on the end of a syringe or placed in a bottle (see Figure 10-6).
  - Commercial supplementer: A thin, flexible tubing leading from a container to the end of the mother's nipple.

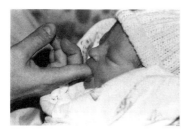

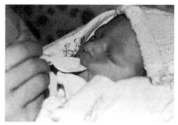

Figure 10-4 Index Finger Inserted Pad Side Up into the Baby's Mouth
Source: Printed with permission of Kay Hoover

Figure 10-5 A Baby Being Fed by a Spoon
Source: Printed with permission of Kay Hoover

- Method:

  - Extend the tubing about one quarter of an inch beyond the end of the nipple.
  - Position the container at a height to produce about one suck per swallow.
  - Threading tubing through the pad part of a bandaid placed on the breast will keep it in place.
  - Check the baby's mouth to make sure tubing is not irritating the roof of the mouth.
  - After every use, flush the tubing with cold water, wash with hot soapy water, and rinse with clear water.

Cup Feeding (See Figure 10-7)

- Considerations:

  - Less invasive to a baby's oral cavity than finger feeding or an artificial nipple
  - Provides sensory stimulus of the lips, olfactory senses, and tongue
  - Helps the baby learn to extend the tongue over the alveolar ridge
  - Promotes appropriate tongue movement used during breastfeeding
  - The baby can pace intake and swallowing occurs when the baby is ready.

- Method:

  - Fill the cup about half way.
  - Hold the baby in a semisitting position.
  - Bring the cup to the baby's lips, resting the rim on the lower lip so it touches the corners of the mouth.
  - Tip the cup until milk touches the baby's lips so the baby can lap the milk.
  - The baby's tongue forms a trough as in breastfeeding.

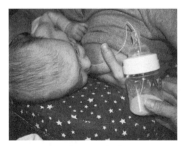

Figure 10-6 Baby Breastfeeding with a Homemade Supplementer Using a Bottle and Tubing
Source: Printed with permission of Anna Swisher

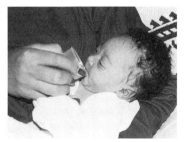

Figure 10-7 A Baby Being Fed by a Cup
Source: Printed with permission of Kay Hoover

- Precautions:
    - The baby does not get practice suckling.
    - Spillage occurs.
    - Pouring milk directly into the baby's mouth increases the risk of aspiration.
    - Slow pacing is important for avoiding aspiration.
    - The time required for feedings may result in noncompliance and eventual bottle use.

Finger Feeding with Tubing (See Figure 10-8)

- Considerations:

    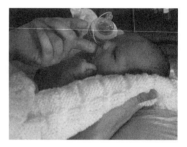

    - More invasive than a lactation aid at the breast or cup feeding
    - The baby may imprint to the finger and prefer it to the breast.
    - Finger feeding can help a baby with low muscle tone or an absent or disorganized suck.

- Method:

    Figure 10-8 Baby Being Finger Fed with Tubing Attached to the Mother's Finger
    Source: Printed with permission of Anna Swisherr

    - Insert number 5, 6, or 8 French oral gastric tubing on the end of a syringe or in a bottle.
    - Prime the tubing with the milk and crimp it to stop the flow until it is in position.
    - Position container height to produce about one suck per swallow.
    - Place the other end of the tubing on the pad side of the caregiver or parent's finger.
    - Hold the baby in an upright or semiupright position.
    - Gently tickle the baby's lips to encourage the mouth to open and invite the finger.
    - Place the fat pad of the finger into the baby's mouth against the soft palate and uncrimp the tubing to allow milk flow.

- Precautions:

    - Ensure that the finger nail is short and smooth.
    - Be sure the baby is at a 45° angle to avoid milk getting into the ears.
    - More than four sucks per swallow may be tiring to the baby.
    - Check the baby's mouth to make sure tubing is not irritating the roof of the mouth.
    - After every use, flush the tubing with cold water, wash with hot soapy water, and rinse with clear water.

Bottle Feeding

- Bottle and nipple choice:

  - Select a nipple with a large base to encourage a wide, open mouth.
  - If smacking or clicking occurs, try a different nipple.
  - Use silicone rather than latex nipples.
  - Select a bottle that is easy to clean and hold comfortably.

- Feeding technique:

  - Respond to feeding behavior.

    ‣ Hold the baby at a 45° angle, with the baby's head positioned higher than the stomach.
    ‣ Swaddling may help prevent the baby's arms from flailing.
    ‣ Support the baby's neck, shoulders, back, and torso.
    ‣ Touch the corner of the baby's mouth to stimulate sucking.

  - Allow the baby to root for the nipple.

    ‣ Tickle the baby's upper lip with the nipple, and let the baby pull in the nipple over the tongue.
    ‣ Hold the bottle at a horizontal angle to prevent rapid flow and so the baby's neck angles up for a clear airway.

  - Pace the feeding.

    ‣ Remove the bottle after two or three sucks to promote a suck–swallow–breathe pattern.
    ‣ Put the bottle back to the baby's mouth for another cycle, and continue this pattern for the entire feeding.

  - Avoid overstimulation from a rocking motion or stress from constantly moving the nipple in the baby's mouth.

- Simulating breastfeeding with bottle feeding:

  - Hold the baby alternately in the right and left arms.
  - Provide frequent skin-to-skin contact.
  - Cuddle the baby for 15 to 20 minutes after the feeding.
  - Give the baby a pacifier for nonnutritive sucking.

- Precautions:

  - Long-term use of a bottle nipple can weaken the baby's suck and contribute to malocclusion.
  - The baby must protect an airway by clamping down on the nipple to stop flow.
  - If the baby attempts to swallow and breathe at the same time, milk may be aspirated.

- A baby who gulps down a full bottle quickly is attempting to breathe.
- Observe the baby for signs of stress.
- Refer to the baby's caregiver if:

  ▶ The baby cannot sustain sucking on a bottle.
  ▶ Milk leaks from the baby's mouth.
  ▶ There is no "pop" sound when the bottle is removed.

Tutorial for Students and Interns

Key Clinical Management Strategies

From *Clinical Guidelines for the Establishment of Exclusive Breastfeeding*, ILCA, 2005.

- If medically indicated, provide additional nutrition using a method of supplementation that is least likely to compromise transition to exclusive breastfeeding.
- Avoid using pacifiers, artificial nipples, and supplements, unless medically indicated.

Key Clinical Competencies

From *Clinical Competencies for IBCLC Practice* available at www.iblce.org.

- Assist mothers with continuation of breastfeeding when the mother is separated from her baby.
- Assist mothers with milk expression techniques.
- Assist mothers with collection, storage, and transportation of milk.
- Assist mothers with safe formula preparation and feeding techniques.
- Assist mothers with induced lactation and relactation.
- Use breastfeeding equipment appropriately and provide information about risks as well as benefits of products, maintaining an awareness of conflict of interest if profiting from the rental or sale of breastfeeding equipment.
- Instruct the mother about avoidance of early use of a pacifier and bottle nipple.
- Demonstrate appropriate use and understanding of potential disadvantages or risks of:

  - A device to evert nipples
  - Nipple creams and ointments
  - Breast shells
  - Breast pumps
  - Spoon feeding
  - Cup feeding
  - Tube feeding at the breast
  - Eyedropper feeding

- Finger feeding
- Bottles and artificial nipples
- Nipple shields
- Pacifiers
- Infant scales

From Theory to Practice
Techniques and Devices

1. Under what circumstances would you suggest that a mother perform a pinch test on her nipples?
2. What is the difference between breast massage and breast compression?
3. Under what circumstances would you suggest reverse pressure softening to a mother?
4. When can a mother discontinue supporting her breast during feeds?
5. When would the Dancer hand position be helpful for a feeding session?
6. How would you teach the technique of hand expression to a mother?
7. What is the reasoning behind recommending that a mother alternate hand expression between breasts two or three times during a session?
8. What would you teach mothers about the use of lubricants on the nipple or breast? When are they appropriate?
9. What is the purpose of inverting a syringe for use on the breast? What alternative techniques are available?
10. In what circumstances are breast shells helpful to a mother?
11. What are appropriate reasons for a mother to use a nipple shield?
12. What are the potential risks of giving a nipple shield to a mother? What can you do to minimize the risks?
13. What is the proper procedure for using a nipple shield?
14. For what reasons other than establishing, increasing, or maintaining milk production would a mother use a breast pump?
15. How would regular milk expression between feedings affect the amount of milk available to the baby during a feeding?
16. How would you respond to a mother who is discouraged by the small amount of milk she is able to pump?
17. When is a handheld breast pump sufficient rather than a double electric pump?
18. A mother tells you she would like to give her baby a pacifier during his fussy period every evening. She is concerned that it could affect his breastfeeding. How would you approach helping her? What would be your first statement to her?
19. What techniques would you routinely teach to all mothers? Why?

Alternate Feeding Methods

1. Under what circumstances would spoon feeding be the most appropriate method for feeding a mother's milk to her baby?
2. What makes tube feeding at the breast a preferred method for supplementing a baby?
3. What precautions are associated with tube feeding?
4. When would it be more appropriate to use cup feeding than tube feeding at the breast?
5. In what circumstance is finger feeding a useful tool?
6. Why is flexible tubing preferred over a periodontal syringe for finger feeding?
7. What are the drawbacks to finger feeding?
8. If a mother asks what kind of nipple she should use for an occasional bottle how would you respond?
9. What might cause a smacking or clicking noise when sucking on an artificial nipple?
10. Why is it recommended that a mother pace her baby's feeding when using a bottle?
11. How can a mother help control the rate of flow with bottle feeding?
12. How can a bottle-fed baby receive some of the same nurturing benefits as those of a breastfed baby?
13. What would cause a baby to become stressed while being bottle fed?
14. What are the concerns about long-term effects of bottle feeding?

CHAPTER 11

Special Situations

In This Chapter

Maternal Health Conditions

Autoimmune Disorders

- The immune system misfires and attacks the cells, tissues, or organs it normally protects.

  - There are more than 80 autoimmune diseases. Many share common symptoms, and often more than one is present.
  - Symptoms usually are present for several years before correct diagnosis.
  - Autoimmune disorders strike three times as many women as men, and genetic predisposition causes clusters in families. Women are most vulnerable during their reproductive years.
  - Human milk has protective factors that reduce the risk of autoimmune diseases.

- Autoimmune issues related to pregnancy:

  - Endometriosis is associated with a higher incidence of autoimmune disorders than the general female population; 41% of women with endometriosis have fertility problems.
  - Multiple sclerosis may improve during pregnancy.
  - Lupus worsens during pregnancy and may improve afterward.
  - Thyroid diseases increase the risk of infertility.

- Counseling implications:

  - Be alert to symptoms such as chronic fatigue and pain, and recommend that the mother consult a caregiver experienced with autoimmune disease.
  - Be alert to potential symptoms that could affect lactation.

    - Chronic fatigue and pain can affect coping abilities and mental outlook (serotonin reuptake inhibitors relieve symptoms for some of the diseases).
    - Sjögren's syndrome impairs the ability of secretory glands to produce moisture, which could potentially have implications for milk production (though this has not been studied).

> Autoimmune disorders most familiar to the general public:
>
> ▶ Multiple sclerosis
> ▶ Graves' disease
> ▶ Scleroderma
> ▶ Raynaud's phenomenon
> ▶ Inflammatory bowel disease
> ▶ Ulcerative colitis
> ▶ Crohn's disease
> ▶ Lupus
> ▶ Sjögren's syndrome
> ▶ Rheumatoid arthritis
> ▶ Fibromyalgia
> ▶ Chronic fatigue

Raynaud's Phenomenon

- Blood flow in the extremities is restricted when exposed to cold.

  - Raynaud's affects up to 22% of women aged 21 to 50.
  - Stress (as in during birth) can cause vasoconstriction even without exposure to cold.

- Symptoms:

  - Numbness and pins and needles sensations
  - Dull pain and clumsiness, which could affect dexterity and ability to relax during a feeding
  - Skin color changes in a sequence:

    - White (blanching or pallor)
    - Blue (cyanotic)
    - Red (rubor) as blood returns to the area

- Causes:

  - Poor latch that compresses the nipple
  - Injury such as frostbite or surgery
  - Regular use of machinery that vibrates; frequent typing or piano playing
  - Causes of secondary Raynaud's:

    - Certain drugs such as heart, blood, and migraine headache medications
    - Scleroderma, a thickening and hardening of the skin and other body tissues

- Systemic lupus erythematosus, a chronic inflammation of the skin and organ systems
- Rheumatoid arthritis, a chronic inflammation and swelling of tissue in the joints
- Problems that slow or stop blood flow in a vessel, such as arteriosclerosis, inflammation, and hardening of the arteries
- Problems that affect the nerves supplying the muscles
- Pulmonary hypertension, a condition in which blood pressure rises in the blood vessels of the lungs

• A Raynaud-like phenomenon can cause vasospasms of the nipple.

  ▪ A stinging, tingling, burning, very painful sensation persists after the feeding.
  ▪ The same triphasic color change occurs as with true Raynaud's.
  ▪ Nipple pain can occur with exposure to cold.

• Dietary counseling:

  ▪ Limit caffeine and nicotine, which increase the severity of Raynaud's.
  ▪ Increasing intake of vitamin B_6 has helped some mothers.

    - Very high doses (600 mg) can lower milk production.
    - Vitamin B_6 passes readily into mothers' milk, and too much can harm an infant's liver.
    - Hale suggests a maximum intake of 25 mg/day of vitamin B_6.

  ▪ Calcium channel blockers, such as nifedipine, have helped some mothers.

• Comfort measures:

  ▪ Apply heat immediately after breastfeeding to minimize the vasospasm.
  ▪ Protect the entire body from cold, not just the hands and feet.
  ▪ Avoid putting hands in cold water.
  ▪ Remove food from the refrigerator or freezer with gloves and potholders.
  ▪ Avoid cuts, bruises, and other injuries to the affected areas.
  ▪ Limit activities such as typing, sewing, or other fine detail work.

Diabetes Mellitus

• Insulin production is insufficient or use of insulin by the body's cells is inefficient.

  ▪ The body is unable to metabolize carbohydrates and burns fat as its energy source.
  ▪ Increased amounts of ketones are excreted into the urine.
  ▪ Uncontrolled blood sugar levels can lead to coma.

SPECIAL SITUATIONS

- Classifications of diabetes:

  - Insulin-dependent (IDDM): Women may breastfeed safely and continue insulin therapy.
  - Non-insulin-dependent (NIDDM): Diet-controlled diabetic women have no breastfeeding restrictions. Pregnant women usually switch from oral hypoglycemic agents to insulin.
  - Gestational (GDM): Gestational diabetes disappears following delivery. Lactogenesis II may be delayed.
  - Some women have insulin resistance rather than full-fledged diabetes, identified by:

    - High weight gain in pregnancy or preexisting obesity
    - Gestational diabetes
    - High cholesterol
    - Hypertension
    - Acanthosis nigricans
    - Development of skin tags during pregnancy

- Fluctuations can occur postpartum.

  - Insulin needs drop dramatically after the delivery of the placenta.
  - Insulin levels fluctuate erratically while lactation is established and with weaning.

    - The mother may need to adjust her insulin dosage.
    - The mother may experience a remission throughout lactation.

      - Hormone balance is altered.
      - Sugar is absorbed for milk production.
      - Breastfeeding expends several hundred calories daily.
      - Remission may permit higher caloric intake and lower insulin dosage.

- The mother's needs related to lactation:

  - Lactogenesis II is delayed by up to 2 to 3 days.
  - The mother may have better diabetic control during lactation than at other times.
  - Mothers generally require an increase in calories, carbohydrates, and protein.
  - Infection or stress can disturb the balance of diet, insulin, and exercise.
  - Diabetic women are prone to yeast infection.

- Blood sugar levels need tight control.

  - High blood sugar releases acetone and transmits it to the baby through the milk.

    - With continued exposure to high acetone, the baby can develop an enlarged liver.
    - Increased carbohydrates and insulin will control acetone risk.

- With low blood sugar, diabetic shock could release epinephrine and inhibit milk production and release.
- The mother must monitor her blood sugar if she has mastitis, has an interruption in breastfeeding, is weaning, or finds sugar present in her urine.

Insufficient Milk Supply (IMS)

- Markers for insufficient milk supply:

    - Shape, symmetry, and vein prominence in the breasts
    - Minimal breast growth during puberty and pregnancy
    - Minimal breast fullness or engorgement after delivery
    - Soft, flaccid, or lumpy and knotty breasts
    - Hypoplasia and intramammary spacing greater than 1.5 inches

- Delay in lactogenesis:

    - Cesarean delivery
    - Hypertension
    - Edema
    - Birth control
    - Diabetes
    - Retained placenta
    - Obesity
    - Theca lutein cyst

- Secondary lactation failure:

    - Scheduled or infrequent feedings
    - Maternal medications, birth control, or herbs
    - Premature infant
    - Ineffective latch or suck
    - Infant ankyloglossia

- Disorders associated with insufficient milk supply:

    - Infertility
    - Thyroid disorders
    - Miscarriage
    - Polycystic ovarian syndrome (PCOS)

- Medications that may help with IMS:

    - Natural progesterone
    - Metoclopramide
    - Domperidone
    - Metformin

SPECIAL SITUATIONS

Polycystic Ovarian Syndrome (PCOS)

- PCOS is the leading cause of infertility in women and is associated with accumulation of incompletely developed follicles in the ovaries.
- Typical symptoms of PCOS:

  - Irregular menstrual cycles
  - Scanty or absent menses
  - Multiple small ovarian cysts
  - Mild to severe hirsutism (excessive hair)
  - Infertility
  - Diabetes with insulin resistance
  - Prolactin resistance, a possible explanation for alactogenesis (no onset of lactogenesis II)

- Improving insulin resistance may help increase milk production.

  - Treating women prenatally may improve outcomes. If treated with medication prenatally, the mother may need to continue the medication after delivery for improved milk production.
  - Outcomes for women with PCOS:

    ‣ Some breastfeed easily.
    ‣ Some experience oversupply of milk, especially multiparas.
    ‣ Some experience undersupply.

Thyroid Disorders

- Thyroid disorders are very common.

  - Rates of miscarriage, fetal death, and cognitive deficits in babies are higher.
  - Pregnant women need close monitoring when they have thyroid therapy.

- Hypothyroidism results from a deficiency in thyroid secretion.

  - Symptoms include sluggishness, low blood pressure, dry skin, obesity, and cold sensitivity.
  - A mother receiving thyroid supplementation may breastfeed with no risk to her baby. High dosages can mask latent hypothyroidism in the baby while being breastfed.
  - A baby with latent hypothyroidism could suffer neurological damage after weaning.
  - There may be a link between untreated hypothyroidism and insufficient milk supply.

- A goiter is enlargement of the thyroid gland resulting from insufficient iodine.

  - It results in a thick looking neck or double-chin appearance.

- Untreated goiters have no impact on breastmilk iodine.
- The mother can increase iodine intake with iodine rich foods or supplements.

- Hyperthyroidism results when the thyroid produces too much thyroid hormone.

  - Graves disease, a form of hyperthyroidism, results in a staring, wide-eyed appearance.
  - Treatment with methimazole is compatible with breastfeeding.
  - Only small amounts of propylthiouracil (PTU) secrete into breastmilk.

- With postpartum thyroiditis (PPT), thyroid function fluctuates, resulting in transient hyperthyroidism or hypothyroidism.

  - It usually resolves within a year after birth.
  - There is a higher prevalence among insulin-dependent diabetics.

Cystic Fibrosis

- Cystic fibrosis is an inherited disease that affects the exocrine system and causes mucus, sweat, saliva, and digestive juices to be thick and sticky, clogging ducts and tubes throughout the body.
- There may be a higher rate of miscarriage, preterm births, and perinatal death.
- Breastfeeding is possible with careful attention to the mother's nutritional requirements.
- Adults with cystic fibrosis are at increased risk for diabetes.
- Lymphocytes in breastmilk become sensitized to pathogens and protect the baby.
- Macronutrients in milk decrease during lung infections, requiring monitoring.
- Average breastfeeding duration is less than 3 months.

Maternal Phenylketonuria (PKU)

- Maternal PKU is a rare inherited disease that can cause brain damage unless treated immediately after birth.
- A woman who had PKU as an infant requires a special PKU diet during pregnancy.
- Maternal phenylalanine overload would affect the growing brain of the fetus.
- Breastfeeding can occur safely with special diets before conception and during pregnancy.

Tuberculosis

- Tuberculosis is a bacterial disease that attacks the lungs and other body parts.
- Breast tuberculosis is rare and seen mostly in developing countries.
- A mother with active tuberculosis may breastfeed with precautions.

SPECIAL SITUATIONS

- When discovered before birth, treatment must begin immediately during pregnancy and infant prophylaxis must begin at birth.
- When discovered postpartum, all contact between the mother and infant, including breastfeeding, must be suspended until after 2 weeks of therapy.

Hepatitis C

- There is no evidence that breastfeeding transmits hepatitis C to the baby.
- Human milk, even if it contains the virus, does not cause infection in newborns.

Herpes

- Varicella zoster and herpes simplex begin as small red pimples that develop into fluid-filled blisters, which dry up and heal.

  - Exposure to active herpes lesions can be fatal to a neonate.
  - All active lesions must be covered to prevent exposure.
  - Breastfeeding is acceptable if active lesions are covered.
  - If a lesion is present on the nipple, the mother cannot breastfeed or feed her milk to her infant from that breast until the lesion heals.

- Epstein-Barr (infectious mononucleosis) presents no threat to the breastfeeding infant.
- Varicella zoster (shingles and chickenpox) is contracted through direct contact or through droplets from the nose or mouth.

  - If the mother is infected at the time of delivery:

    - She must be isolated from her infant until the lesions heal completely.
    - She can feed her milk to her infant if there are no lesions on her breast.

  - A mother who is infected up to 7 days before delivery or up to 28 days after delivery must receive zoster immunoglobulin (ZIG).
  - A lactating mother who is infected should continue to breastfeed.

- Herpes simplex is contracted through direct exposure to the lesions.

  - The infection can be present in the infant without any maternal history.
  - Herpes simplex I (cold sore or fever blister) usually appears on the mouth and nose areas.
  - Herpes simplex II (genitalis) is usually transmitted through sexual contact.
  - Neonates contract the disease through direct contact with infected tissue.
  - Mortality rates are high for infants exposed to herpes genitalis during vaginal birth.

- Cytomegalovirus (CMV), when contracted in early infancy, is usually contracted from the infant's mother.

- Symptoms include fatigue, fever, swollen lymph glands, pneumonia, and liver or spleen defects.
- The breast is the most frequent site of CMV reactivation in postpartum women.
- Excretion of CMV in the mother's milk seems to peak after 2 to 12 weeks.
- Term infants can breastfeed even when the mother is shedding the virus in her milk.
- Babies may receive passive immunity to CMV through their mothers' milk.
- Danger to the infant is the possibility of seroconversion if the infant of a seronegative mother receives donor milk from a seropositive mother.
- CMV is especially dangerous for premature infants or infants who are immunologically impaired.
- Pasteurization at 62°C for 8 minutes can destroy CMV in human milk.

Human Immunodeficiency Virus (HIV)

- HIV, a retrovirus that destroys the human immune system, can lead to acquired immune deficiency syndrome (AIDS).

- Route of transmission:

  - Through sexual contact, contaminated blood, and intravenous drug use
  - From mother to infant during pregnancy, delivery, and (it is believed) breastfeeding

- Breastfeeding issues:

  - Most breastfed infants remain uninfected, despite prolonged and repeated exposure.
  - Human milk may provide some protection to the infant.
  - Pasteurization inactivates HIV in breastmilk (at 56 to 62.5°C for 12 to 15 minutes).
  - Avoid breastfeeding when replacement feeding is acceptable, feasible, affordable, sustainable, and safe.
  - Breastfeed exclusively with early and rapid weaning at around 4 to 6 months of age when replacement feeding is not acceptable, feasible, affordable, sustainable, and safe.

> **ADVICE TO CLINICIANS**
> **TEACH MOTHERS**
>
> That during illness or hospitalization:
>
> ▸ Pump to maintain milk production.
> ▸ Decrease the baby's exposure by careful hand washing before contact.
> ▸ Have another adult in the room to help the mother care for her baby.
> ▸ Have the baby brought to the hospital throughout the day to breastfeed.
> ▸ Nurse before and after surgery.

Maternal Conditions that Contraindicate Breastfeeding

- Sheehan's syndrome prevents the mother from producing milk.
- Some long-term drug therapies are dangerous to infants.
- Severe illness in the mother may contraindicate breastfeeding.
- Women with unresolved congestive heart failure or on chemotherapy treatment for cancer should not breastfeed.
- Active tuberculosis requires 2 weeks of temporary weaning.
- Women who test positive for HIV and live in a developed country with sanitary water should not breastfeed.

Infant Health Conditions

Phenylketonuria (PKU)

- PKU is a genetic disease in which an infant lacks an enzyme needed to change phenylalanine, an amino acid in food protein, into a form the body can use.

  - Phenylalanine intake must be restricted, with strict monitoring.
  - The physician may interrupt breastfeeding to stabilize phenylalanine levels and determine the appropriate diet.

- Needs of a breastfed baby with PKU:

  - Daily intake of 20 ounces of human milk supplemented with phenylalanine-free formula.
  - Vitamin and mineral supplements, which are absent in phenylalanine-free formula.
  - Minimal fluid requirements because of the lower solute load of human milk.

- Managing feedings:

  - Periodic test weighing will track the amount of breastmilk consumed.
  - Breastfeeding can be adapted to the baby's phenylalanine blood concentrations.
  - Feeding options:

    ▸ Breastfeed at each feeding until the baby is satiated to ensure both foremilk and hindmilk. Feed phenylalanine-free formula within 15 minutes after breastfeeding, or through a tube-feeding device at the breast.
    ▸ Alternate feedings between breastfeeding and phenylalanine-free bottle feeding.

  - If phenylalanine levels are high:

    ▸ Pump milk from the breasts before breastfeeding.
    ▸ Feed the phenylalanine-free formula and then put the baby to breast.

> ▶ Use a tube-feeding device while the baby nurses on a breast she just pumped.

- Diagnosis is reconfirmed between 3 and 12 months of age.

  > ▶ The baby receives a phenylalanine load for 3 days, in cow's milk or formula.
  > ▶ If the mother continues to breastfeed, phenylalanine content of her milk must be measured.

- Dietary changes:
  - Evaluating energy content of the milk will determine if a dietary change is required.
  - Weaning may occur early if it is difficult to control the baby's phenylalanine levels.
  - Weaning requires close monitoring to maintain balance.

    > ▶ Replace each dropped feeding with the correct amount of phenylalanine-free or low-phenylalanine formula or solid foods.
    > ▶ Designate a target date and estimate what the baby's weight will be.
    > ▶ Determine the baby's requirements for phenylalanine, protein, and energy at that time.
    > ▶ Calculate amounts of phenylalanine-free or low-phenylalanine formula and other supplements needed.

Galactosemia

- Galactosemia is an inherited disease in which the liver enzyme that changes galactose to glucose is absent.

ADVICE TO CLINICIANS
SUPPORT MOTHERS

Tips for mothers of babies with special health needs:

- ▶ Help parents deal with emotions and stages of grief for the "perfect" child.
- ▶ Avoid comments that minimize parents' concerns or deny their reactions.
- ▶ Give parents information in gradual doses during the newborn period.
- ▶ Help parents view their child as normal in other respects.
- ▶ Avoid evaluating or judging their breastfeeding.
- ▶ Help the mother with pumping and provide follow-up care after discharge home.
- ▶ Teach parents coping mechanisms and refer to specialists.

SPECIAL SITUATIONS

- An infant with galactosemia is unable to metabolize lactose and cannot breastfeed.

Cleft Defects

- The upper lip and/or palate fail to fuse during the first trimester of pregnancy.

  - A cleft in the palate produces an opening to the nasal cavity.
  - A cleft can occur as part of other congenital anomalies, syndromes, and medical complications.
  - A submucosal cleft palate can escape newborn screening because a layer of skin covers a cleft in the soft palate. Markers include:

    - Bluish midline discoloration
    - Drooling
    - Bifid (forked) uvula
    - A short, soft palate with a furrow in the midline
    - A bony notch in the posterior of the hard palate

  - Pierre Robin sequence (syndrome) is a rare anomaly that occurs with a cleft palate.

    - The syndrome includes a receding lower jaw, displacement at the back of the tongue, and an absence of the gag reflex (see Figure 11-1).
    - Possible severity of airway obstruction and concerns over survival usually make direct breastfeeding unlikely, though an infant with a very slight case may be able to breastfeed.

- Surgical repair:

  - Lip repair usually occurs by 3 months of age.
  - The baby may resume breastfeeding immediately following lip repair surgery.
  - Palatal growth determines when palatal repair occurs.

- Breastfeeding issues:

  - A cleft can affect the infant's ability to generate suction and obtain adequate nourishment.
  - Multiparas may establish milk production better initially than primiparas.
  - An isolated cleft lip presents no physiologic impediment to breastfeeding.

    - Breast tissue can fill the cleft to seal it.
    - The mother can place her thumb over the cleft to improve the seal.

  - A cleft palate prevents the baby from creating a vacuum and holding the breast in his or her mouth.

> ‣ The mother can cup her breast as she brings her baby toward her to latch on, and maintain hold throughout the feeding.
> ‣ Milk transfer may be easiest at the beginning of a feeding when the breast is firmer.
> ‣ Breast massage before and during the feed will help the baby transfer milk.
> ‣ Short, frequent feedings will prevent the infant from tiring. Put the baby to breast at least every 2 hours in the newborn period.

- ▪ Positioning and latch:

> ‣ Hold the baby upright, with the nose and throat higher than the breast to minimize milk leaking into the nasal cavity.
> ‣ Push the baby's chin to his or her chest to stop choking and then resume feeding.
> ‣ The baby can be held upright straddling the mother's body, or be held in the football position.
> ‣ With a unilateral cleft, the breast enters on the side of the cleft so the infant's cheek on the side of the defect touches the breast.
> ‣ With a bilateral cleft, the breast enters at midline.
> ‣ An obturator placed over a cleft in the palate will assist in feeding until repair (see Figure 11-2).

- ▪ Breast pumping maintains milk production.

> ‣ Makes milk readily available at the beginning of a feeding.
> ‣ Removes milk after a feeding.

- ▪ Specialty bottles are available for feeding babies with a cleft palate.

- • Support for the parents

  - ▪ Parents have a range of reactions.

> ‣ Visibility of an unrepaired cleft lip leads to an immediate emotional response.

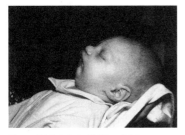

Figure 11-1 Infant with Pierre Robin Sequence
Source: Printed with permission of Linda Kutner

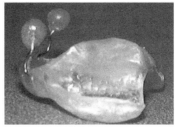

Figure 11-2 Obturator
Source: Printed with permission of Dr. Scott Franklin

> ‣ Comment on how well the mother is doing in her maternal role.
> ‣ Comment on the baby's positive attributes.
> ‣ Avoid comments that minimize the parents' concerns or deny the mother's reactions.
> ‣ Avoid implying that surgery will completely conceal a cleft; traces will remain.

- Give parents information in gradual doses, and repeat facts as they progress.

  > ‣ Help them anticipate difficulties in feeding and care.
  > ‣ They need to know signs and symptoms of illness and possible complications.
  > ‣ Help them learn how to deal with reactions of friends and family.
  > ‣ Help them view their child as normal in other respects.

- Avoid judging their breastfeeding experience. Validate the mother's disappointment if she weans early or does not breastfeed.

Spina Bifida

- Spina bifida is a common congenital nerve defect that results in a gap in the bone that surrounds the spinal cord.
- It causes weakness or paralysis of the lower extremities.
- The baby can go to breast as soon as it is allowable after repair.
- Positioning needs to avoid pressure on the baby's spinal column.
- Feeding times will be brief during recovery, which may take several weeks.

ADVICE TO CLINICIANS
TEACH MOTHERS

Tips for mothers of a compromised infant:

▸ Put the newborn to breast on cue and with great frequency (at least every 2 hours).
▸ Hold the baby upright with his or her nose and throat higher than the breast.
▸ Provide skin-to-skin contact.
▸ Begin a feeding before the baby is completely awake.
▸ Nurse for brief periods and more frequently to avoid tiring the baby.
▸ Recognize signs of fatigue, cardiac complications, hypotonia, and difficulty rooting and sucking.
▸ View early breastfeeds as practice sessions.
▸ Press down on the center of the tongue, and use the Dancer hand position to assist the baby as needed.

Down Syndrome

- Down syndrome is a congenital anomaly caused by the presence of an extra chromosome.
- Markers include:

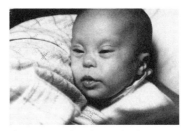

Figure 11-3 Baby with Down Syndrome
Source: Printed with permission of Sarah Coulter Danner

  - Oval eyes that slant slightly upward (see Figure 11-3)
  - A protruding tongue that seems too large for the mouth
  - Short stature, small ears, and a wide, flattened nose
  - Muscular weakness and hypotonicity (low muscle tone)

- Most babies with Down syndrome are able to breastfeed.

  - Rooting and sucking may be difficult because of weak reflexes.
  - The baby may be sluggish and become easily fatigued at the breast.
  - Watch for signs of fatigue, which makes it difficult to transfer milk.
  - Muscle tone improves as the baby learns to exercise and stretch his or her muscles.

- Maximize the baby's position for feedings.

  - Support the baby's head and body well to minimize the effort required.
  - Position the baby's throat slightly above the level of the nipple to prevent choking and gagging.
  - In the side-lying position, support the baby with several pillows and prop the head higher than the rest of the body.
  - The football hold gives the mother more ability to form and control her breast.

- Assist the baby's latch.

  - Press down on the chin to help the baby's mouth to open.
  - Check that the bottom lip turns outward over the alveolar ridge.
  - Press down on the center of the tongue several times before feeding to help the baby learn to shape the tongue appropriately.
  - Use the Dancer hand position during the feeding.

- Assist milk transfer.

  - Massage and express milk to initiate letdown before putting the baby to breast.
  - Initiate feedings frequently, nursing for 10 to 12 minutes on each breast every 2 to 3 hours.
  - Observe the baby for subtle signs of wakefulness and readiness to feed.
  - Express milk after feeding to obtain hindmilk to feed to the baby.

Hydrocephalus

- Excessive accumulation of cerebrospinal fluid in the intracranial cavity causes the head to enlarge.
- Hydrocephalus results from interference in the flow or absorption of fluid through the brain and the spinal canal.
- The baby usually has a high-pitched cry, muscle weakness, and severe neurological defects.
- Breastfeeding is possible with the baby's head slightly higher than the breast and with frequent feedings to avoid reflux.

Neurological Impairment

- The infant rarely has a fully developed or strong suck and swallow reflex.
- A severely impaired infant is unable to maintain concentration.

  - The brain does not pick up the impetus to perform specific functions.
  - The infant forgets reflexes that were instinctive at birth and must be taught.
  - He forgets learned abilities and requires continual reinforcement.
  - He may not have the ability to coordinate reflexes with the stimulus.
  - He may have difficulty swallowing, resulting in gagging and choking.

- The baby may continually forget how to nurse and require coaxing.

  - Nurse in an upright position.
  - Stroke downward under the chin to aid swallowing.
  - Feed for brief 5-minute periods and more frequently.
  - Express milk to initiate letdown before putting the baby to breast.

Sensory Processing Disorder

- With low registration of sensory input (hyporesponsive), the baby may fail to suckle when put to the breast.

  - Finger feed to pattern suckling.
  - Gently massage the baby's face, mouth, and palate.
  - Hold the baby upright for feeding.

- With high registration of input (hyperresponsive), the baby may be hypertonic, easily overstimulated, and aversive to the breast.

  - Use deep pressure touch when holding the baby.
  - Swaddle the baby.
  - Swing the baby gently from head to toe in a blanket before feeding.
  - Allow the baby to self-attach.

Tutorial for Students and Interns

Key Clinical Management Strategies

From *Clinical Guidelines for the Establishment of Exclusive Breastfeeding*, ILCA, 2005.

- Identify maternal and infant risk factors that may affect the mother's or infant's ability to breastfeed effectively, and provide appropriate assistance and follow-up.
- Support exclusive breastfeeding during any illness or hospitalization of mother or infant.
- Identify any maternal and infant contraindications to breastfeeding.

Key Clinical Competencies

From *Clinical Competencies for IBCLC Practice* available at www.iblce.org.

- Assist mothers with maintaining milk production.
- Assist mothers with overproduction of milk.
- Identify situations in which immediate verbal communication with the healthcare provider is necessary, such as serious illness in the infant, child, or mother.
- Assist mothers with neurodevelopmental problems.
- Assist mothers with chronic medical conditions, such as multiple sclerosis, lupus, and seizures.
- Assist mothers with disabilities that may limit a mother's ability to handle the baby easily, such as rheumatoid arthritis, carpal tunnel syndrome, and cerebral palsy.
- Assist mothers with HIV/AIDS in understanding current recommendations.
- Assist mothers with an infant with craniofacial abnormalities, such as micronathia (receding lower jaw) and cleft lip and/or palate.
- Assist mothers with an infant with Down syndrome.
- Assist mothers with an infant with cardiac problems.
- Assist mothers with an infant with chronic medical conditions such as cystic fibrosis and phenylketonuria (PKU).

From Theory to Practice
Maternal Health

1. In what ways can an autoimmune disorder affect breastfeeding?
2. What special breastfeeding issues might a woman with Raynaud's phenomenon have?
3. What symptoms of nipple pain might cause you to consider a Raynaud-like phenomenon?

4. What can a mother do to minimize the discomfort from Raynaud's?
5. What special precautions must a diabetic woman take for breastfeeding her baby?
6. Under what circumstances will a diabetic mother be unable to breastfeed?
7. What special monitoring, if any, is necessary for the infant of a diabetic woman?
8. What explains why some diabetic women experience a remission during lactation?
9. What are the risks of high acetone levels in the mother's milk, and how can the mother avoid its occurrence?
10. What disorders place a woman at risk for insufficient milk production?
11. What is the difference between a delay in lactogenesis and secondary lactation failure?
12. What will you watch for during a breast assessment to rule out the potential for insufficient milk production?
13. Why does a history of polycystic ovarian syndrome place a woman at risk for insufficient milk production?
14. What is a potential complication for a hypothyroid woman who breastfeeds her baby?
15. What are the potential complications of hyperthyroidism, if any, for breastfeeding?
16. How can a woman with cystic fibrosis guard her health and that of her breastfeeding baby?
17. What implications can PKU in the mother have for breastfeeding?
18. What are the breastfeeding guidelines for a mother with active tuberculosis?
19. What are the breastfeeding guidelines for a mother with hepatitis C?
20. What are the breastfeeding guidelines for each type of herpes?
21. How do breastfeeding guidelines for HIV differ depending on geographic location?
22. In what circumstances is it unsafe for a mother to breastfeed?
23. A mother is admitted to the hospital for emergency gall bladder surgery. She has a 2-month-old baby at home. How can you help her?
24. If a mother's hospitalization causes her to be separated from her baby, what can she do to make the separation go smoothly?

Infant Health

25. What are the potential risks of a mother breastfeeding a baby who has PKU?
26. How can a mother ensure that the health of her PKU baby is not compromised by breastfeeding?
27. Why must a mother carefully monitor weaning her PKU baby from the breast?
28. Why does galactosemia prohibit breastfeeding?

29. What special needs does a mother have when breastfeeding a baby who has a cleft palate? What can she do to assist her baby at feeds?
30. What is the reason that a submucosal cleft palate may be undetected at birth?
31. What symptoms might alert you to the possibility of a submucosal cleft palate?
32. What are the breastfeeding implications for a baby with Pierre Robin syndrome?
33. What positioning would you recommend to the mother of an infant with spina bifida?
34. What does a mother need to be alert to when breastfeeding a baby with Down syndrome?
35. What recommendations for positioning and latch can you give to a mother whose baby has Down syndrome?
36. How can the mother of a baby with Down syndrome assist her baby with milk transfer?
37. What breastfeeding adjustments can accommodate a baby with hydrocephalus?
38. What challenges does a mother have when breastfeeding a baby who is severely brain damaged?
39. How does sensory processing disorder affect a baby's ability to breastfeed?
40. What can a mother do to improve breastfeeding for a baby with sensory processing disorder?

CHAPTER 1 2

Supporting
Extended Breastfeeding

In This Chapter

Infant Development in the First Year

Newborn Reflexes

- Rooting, suckling, grasping, and swallowing enable the infant to obtain food.
- The gag reflex protects the baby from choking when learning to take in food.
- The Moro reflex causes the baby to startle in response to sudden noise.
- The Palmer grasp enables the baby to grasp the parents' fingers.
- Pressure on the soles of the feet elicits Bauer's response.
- The Moro reflex, Palmer grasp, and tonic neck disappear at about 4 months.
- Bauer's response and rooting and suckling reflexes continue to about 9 months.

The Baby's Head and Body Control

- Ability at 3 months:
  - The baby's head can rise from a prone position.
- Abilities at 4 to 5 months:
  - The baby can raise his head higher and hold it for longer periods.

- The baby's head turns toward a voice or movement.
- The baby can rest on his or her forearms.
- The baby can control hand movements and waves and bats at objects.
- The baby's back is rounded, with the head erect when held in a sitting position.

- Abilities at 6 months:

  - The baby can roll over.
  - The baby can grasp desired items and pull them toward the mouth.
  - Tongue movement allows the baby to take solid foods.
  - The baby can pull to a sitting position and sit when propped.

- Abilities at 7 months:

  - The baby can roll over in both directions.
  - The baby can wave goodbye and transfer objects from hand to hand.
  - The baby can sit without being propped.

- Abilities at 8 months:

  - The baby can rise onto his or her hands and knees and rocks back and forth.
  - The baby can use his or her thumb and forefinger to pick up objects (pincer grasp).
  - The baby begins the early stages of crawling.

- Abilities at 9 months:

  - The baby can sit well in a chair and pull into a sitting position.

- Abilities at 10 to 12 months:

  - The baby moves about a room by using tables and chairs for balance while learning to walk.

Sleep Patterns

- Physical development determines when a baby will be able to sleep through the night.
- Ability to sleep for longer periods increases as the central nervous system develops.
- Newborns spend 50% of their time in REM sleep (30% by 6 to 12 months).
- By 3 months, the baby usually has at least one longer rest period and several naps each day.
- Nursing directly before the mother retires may provide 5 or 6 hours of uninterrupted sleep.
- By 8 months, the baby may experience separation anxiety during the night and need to nurse.
- In the second year, the baby needs close physical contact to fall asleep.

The Baby's Social Development

- Development at 3 months:

    - The baby regards him or herself and the mother as one person.
    - The baby responds to stimuli and interacts with the environment.
    - The baby responds to high-pitched voices.
    - The baby is awake for more hours each day and is more alert and responsive.
    - The baby smiles and recognizes the voices of caregivers.
    - The baby can sense tension in a caregiver and responds with fussiness.
    - Eating and sleeping take on a more definite pattern.

- Development at 4 to 5 months:

    - The baby laughs aloud and uses motor skills for self-amusement.

- Development at 6 months:

    - The baby begins babbling, cooing, and squealing.

- Development at 9 months:

    - The baby may experience separation anxiety and cry in anticipation of the mother leaving.
    - The baby may wake at night and cry out for reassurance that the parents are nearby.
    - The baby may react fearfully to strangers.

- Development at 10 to 12 months:

    - The baby is eager to participate in family activities and mealtimes.
    - The baby freely moves away from the mother to explore the environment.
    - The baby learns to express unhappiness, delight, and excitement.
    - The baby may show a preference for his parents, especially the mother.
    - The baby may feel overwhelmed by contact with strangers, separation from the mother, and changes in schedule.
    - Recognition vocabulary increases, and the baby begins experimenting with vocabulary sounds.

Feeding Behavior

- Behavior at 1 month:

    - The baby is efficient at suckling.
    - The baby actively nurses for 15 minutes or more at a feeding.
    - The baby has 8 to 16 feeds per day.

- Behavior at 2 to 3 months:

  - The baby spends less time at feeding.
  - Suckling is more efficient and the baby may self-comfort.
  - The baby has a growth spurt and feeds more frequently.

- Behavior at 4 to 6 months:

  - The baby is noticeably more efficient at suckling.
  - Feedings are shorter and less frequent.
  - Breastfeeding provides security.
  - The baby pats or strokes the breast and pushes away for a better look at the mother or surroundings.

- Behavior at 6 months:

  - Feeding frequency continues to diminish.
  - The longest nursing usually takes place before being put to bed for the night.
  - Complementary foods and greater activity during the day may cause the baby to wake during the night more often to nurse.
  - Teething begins soon, with increased feedings for comfort and reassurance.

- Behavior at 7 to 12 months:

  - The baby seeks to nurse anytime and anywhere.
  - The baby pulls at the mother's clothing.
  - The baby distracts easily and needs a quiet location for uninterrupted feedings.
  - The baby may hold the breast with one or both hands when feeding.
  - The baby will have begun teething.

- Behavior at 10 to 12 months:

  - Feeding frequency and duration are sporadic depending on the baby's mood and activity level.
  - The baby establishes regular meal patterns.
  - The baby increases feedings to seek comfort and reassurance.
  - Renewed outside pressure may lead the mother to consider weaning.

Breastfeeding a Young Baby
Baby Prefers One Breast

- It is common for a baby to display a preference for one breast.

  - The mother's hand preference may inadvertently promote one breast.
  - The baby may dislike the appearance, feel, or smell of one breast.
  - The baby may dislike the taste of the milk in one breast.
  - A plug of thick milk may have broken loose.

- The mother may have engorgement in one breast.
- The baby may have pain from birth on one side of his face, chin, neck, or shoulder.
- In rare cases, the breast may be malignant.

- Encourage the baby to feed at both breasts.

  - Begin with the preferred breast and express milk from the other breast to start the baby on it.
  - Begin with the less preferred breast after obtaining letdown by preexpressing milk.
  - Offer the less preferred breast when the baby is sleepy and less aware.
  - Use a different position so the baby thinks he is on the preferred breast.
  - Express the less preferred breast regularly to relieve discomfort and maintain production.
  - It is possible to feed on one breast for the duration of breastfeeding.

Baby Loses Interest

- Disinterest in nursing occurs commonly at around 7 months.

  - It may happen suddenly or gradually with decreased feedings.

    - The baby is hungry but cannot settle to breastfeed.
    - The baby goes to breast, mouths the nipple, and then acts disinterested or cries.

  - It usually lasts from only a few days to a week but may continue for several weeks.
  - Disinterest is temporary and is not a sign of weaning.

Renewing a baby's interest in breastfeeding

▶ Cleanse the breasts to remove deodorant or lotions; discontinue new brands.
▶ Feed the baby in the presence of other breastfeeding babies.
▶ Feed the baby with an alternate method briefly, and then put him to breast.
▶ Put the baby to breast frequently without pressuring him to nurse.
▶ Massage the breasts and express milk before feedings to promote letdown.
▶ Perform breast compression during feedings to promote milk flow.
▶ Express milk regularly to maintain milk production and prevent engorgement.
▶ Reduce complementary and supplementary foods to rekindle interest in the breast.
▶ Discontinue any soothing methods, including pacifiers.
▶ Determine if the mother is pregnant or taking new medications.
▶ Work out an alternate feeding plan until the phase passes.

- The baby may be in pain.

  - He is teething.

    ▸ Use comfort measures for sore gums.
    ▸ If pain causes biting and the mother reacts, skin contact and carrying the baby in a sling will help to renew trust.

  - He has an ear infection.

    ▸ Nurse in an upright position or with the football hold to take pressure off the baby's ears.
    ▸ Consult a caregiver about decreasing the baby's mucus.

  - He has thrush or another illness.

- The baby may be interested in new objects and people and is distracted easily.

  - Move away from the distraction.
  - End the feeding and resume when the baby is more interested.
  - Shift position so the baby faces the activity.
  - Let the baby play and nurse intermittently at the breast.
  - Make up for missed daytime feedings in the evening or late night.
  - Feed in a quiet, darkened room.

- Other reasons for disinterest:

  - The baby is efficient at nursing and can obtain more milk in a shorter period.
  - The baby sucks on a thumb or other object.
  - The mother is trying to manipulate the feeding schedule to get the baby to sleep at night.
  - Overexertion, tension, poor eating habits, or fatigue cause decreased feeds.
  - Menstruation changes the taste of the milk and the scent of secretions on the skin.

Breastfeeding in Public

- Watch other women breastfeed discreetly.
- Practice discreet breastfeeding in front of a mirror or another person.
- Wear loose-fitting clothing that allows easy access to the breast.
- Place something over the shoulders to help conceal the breast.
- Carry the baby in a sling to allow easy access and additional coverage.
- Plan feeding time into the schedule.
- Feed the baby before he is overly hungry and fusses.
- Plan where to feed before the baby becomes hungry.

  - A corner table or booth in a restaurant
  - A bench next to a wall

- A store dressing room or lounge
- A parked car

Traveling with a Breastfeeding Baby

- A baby between 6 weeks and 6 months of age travels well.

  - The baby has a predictable routine.
  - The baby is not yet eating complementary foods.
  - The baby is not very mobile and usually sleeps when in motion.

- Plan for the trip.

  - Take only essential items, including items to keep the baby amused.
  - A lightweight diaper bag can double as a purse.
  - Take a baby sling for walking.
  - Breastfeed with the baby in a car seat, plan to stop, or feed expressed milk.
  - Plan time into the schedule to accommodate the baby.
  - When traveling by air, request the roomier seat behind the bulkhead.
  - Check the stroller and other equipment with luggage to free the mother to carry the baby.
  - Breastfeed during takeoff and descent to minimize ear discomfort from altitude changes.

Overfeeding a Breastfed Baby

- A baby is considered overweight if he is two categories above weight for height.

  - Normal weight gain is 1 to 2 pounds per month for the first 4 to 5 months.
  - Rapid weight gain should not continue into the second half of the first year.
  - An older baby who often spits up or vomits may be overfed.

- Actions the mother may take:

  - Let the baby suck on his thumb or finger.
  - Nurse at one breast per feeding and allow the baby to suck on the less full breast.
  - Learn other ways to interact with the baby.

Infant Development After One Year
Social and Emotional Development

- The baby may have a renewed fear of strangers between 12 and 15 months.
- Overstimulation or separation anxiety may cause the baby to wake at night.

- Outside interests become more important than breastfeeding.
- Communication and play become increasingly important.
- Interaction with the father increases.
- The baby learns that absent parents will return.

Feeding Behavior

- The baby enjoys drinking from a cup and using a spoon.
- The baby gains as much as 16 pounds in the first year and weight may double after another 3 years.
- Food preferences become better defined.
- The baby eats one balanced meal a day plus two other partial meals and nutritious snacks.
- The mother's milk continues to supply significant calories, vitamins, minerals, and immunity.
- Breastfeeding frequency fluctuates.

Breastfeeding an Older Baby

Teething and Biting

- Teething typically begins between 6 and 8 months of age and can occur anywhere between 4 to 14 months.

  - The gums swell and are irritated.
  - Blood rushes to the gums with sucking, adding to the swelling.

- Signs that the baby is teething:

  - He quickly pulls away from the breast and cries out with pain.
  - He begins waking during the night to seek comfort.
  - He becomes irritable, rubs his jaw or pulls on his ear.
  - He drools more than usual.
  - He has a slight fever and spits up or develops loose stools.

- Comfort measures:

  - Allow the baby to suck on a cooled teething ring.
  - Place ice or a cold cloth on the gums before breastfeeding.
  - Give him hard food such as toast to chew on.
  - Apply an over-the-counter pain reliever or locally acting preparation.

- The baby may clamp down on the breast when teething or falling asleep.

  - He cannot suckle and bite at the same time and probably is not hungry enough to nurse.
  - Watch signs that the feeding is ending.

- Remove the baby when the suck–swallow–breathe rhythm slows.
- If biting occurs in the middle of a feeding, remove the baby for a few minutes.
- If the baby bites a second time during the feeding, end the feeding.

Toddler Breastfeeding

- Encourage mothers to continue to breastfeed beyond 12 months.

  - Babies breastfed beyond 12 months walk and crawl earlier.
  - Satisfying a baby's emotional needs encourages self-reliance.
  - Sucking needs last for several years.
  - Women who breastfeed longer than 12 months are typically older and better educated, exclusively breastfeed longer, and sleep with their baby more frequently.

- Present the concept of breastfeeding beyond infancy gradually.

  - It is an extension of the warm infant–mother relationship.
  - It is comforting when the baby is stressed or injured, feels hurt or shy, or is in a new environment.
  - It is a comforting way to connect with the mother between explorations.
  - It communicates love even when the mother and baby are at odds over behavior.

- Continue to put the child to breast and respond to his or her wishes.

  - Nurse before offering complementary food.
  - Nurse in a quiet place to limit distractions and interruptions.
  - Allow the child to lessen the number of feedings as he or she receives more foods.
  - The child may assume a position that allows him to conveniently view the room.
  - The child may stand or straddle the breasts.

- Help mothers anticipate challenges.

  - Teeth may cause pressure marks until the child learns to hold the breast with his lips.
  - Crumbs or food particles in the child's mouth may irritate the mother's nipples.
  - The child may insist on nursing at inconvenient or embarrassing moments.

    ▸ He may tug at the mother's clothing and fondle her breasts.
    ▸ Use a special name for nursing and feed at certain times or in a special location at home.
    ▸ Stretch intervals by offering a drink or treat before the usual nursing time.

  - Others may oppose breastfeeding an older baby.

    ▸ The baby's father may worry about social and sexual implications or believe the child appears too dependent.

- The mother can avoid nursing in the father's presence.
- Seeing other children nurse may help the father's perspective.

- ❯ If people other than the baby's father are uncomfortable, the mother can nurse discreetly or not nurse when those people are present.
- ❯ If siblings appear resentful, the mother can set aside special time with each child.

Tandem Breastfeeding

- Breastfeeding during pregnancy:

  - Studies suggest:

    - ❯ There are no significant differences in fetal growth.
    - ❯ Fat stores are reduced when there are less than 6 months between pregnancies.
    - ❯ Weight gain is lower for the new baby and mother during pregnancy.

  - Considerations:

    - ❯ The mother may need to consume more energy and nutrients.
    - ❯ If at risk for preterm labor, the mother may need to wean.
    - ❯ Some pregnant women feel nauseated when the older child nurses.
    - ❯ Hormones of pregnancy alter the composition and taste of the mother's milk.
    - ❯ The child may self-wean.
    - ❯ If the baby is under 1 year of age, monitor intake with frequent weight checks and offer supplements if milk supply decreases.

- Breastfeeding siblings:

  - The toddler can position himself at the breast, making simultaneous feeds manageable.
  - The toddler may understand the concepts of waiting to nurse and taking turns.
  - Put the younger baby to the breast first, when milk production and release are greatest.
  - The older child can nurse on the less full breast and obtain less milk.
  - The mother can reserve a breast for each child or alternate breasts daily to equalize nipple stimulation.
  - The toddler's efficient sucking will increase milk production.

    - ❯ A younger baby may choke from strong flow of milk.
    - ❯ Allow the older child to remove some milk before putting the baby to breast.

Foods Other than Breastmilk
Supplementary Feedings

- Supplementary foods are foods other than human milk fed to the infant following or in place of a breastfeeding. They include, in order of preference:

  - The mother's expressed milk
  - Donor human milk
  - Formula if there is no history of allergy

- Offering supplementary food:

  - Delay until the baby establishes breastfeeding, about 3 weeks of age.
  - Limit the amount so as not to interfere with breastfeeding.

    - Begin with about one ounce once or twice a week.
    - Offer when the baby is not fussy or too hungry.

  - Avoid bottles when other feeding methods are possible.

    - Learning to drink from a cup is often easy for breastfeeding babies.
    - The baby's acceptance of a bottle may require several attempts.

  - If supplementary feeding results in a missed breastfeeding:

    - Nurse or express milk just before departing.
    - Express milk while away.
    - Wear a larger bra to avoid pressure on full breasts.
    - Nurse immediately after returning.

  - Supplemental iron:

    - Breastmilk supplies sufficient iron until a healthy, full-term baby's birth weight triples.
    - A preterm infant or infant of an anemic mother may have low iron stores and need a supplement.
    - Lactoferrin in breastmilk increases iron absorption.
    - Supplementing iron too soon interferes with increased iron absorption and disease protection from lactoferrin.

Complementary Feeding

- Complementary foods are new foods added to a growing infant's diet to meet energy and nutrient needs that are not met by breastmilk alone.
- When to introduce complementary foods:

  - Provide exclusive breastmilk until 6 months of age.

- Babies of average birth weight with adequate fetal stores of fat and iron do well on mother's milk alone until about 6 months of age.
- Breastmilk provides calories, vitamins, and minerals in proportions the baby needs.
- Protective factors help prevent allergy and illness.

- Introduce complementary foods when the baby is able to handle them.

    - Neuromuscular development allows for proper chewing and swallowing of nonliquid foods.
    - Intestinal maturation promotes more complete digestion and absorption of other foods.
    - The baby's body handles waste products from solid foods.
    - The baby's immunologic system is functioning.

- Signs of the baby's readiness for complementary foods:

    - Eruption of teeth
    - Ability to sit up
    - Disappearance of the tongue extrusion reflex
    - Improved eye-hand coordination
    - Ability to grasp objects with the thumb and forefinger
    - Showing interest when others are eating
    - Intensified demand to nurse that is not satisfied after several days of increased breastfeedings. This occurs before 6 months in some babies.

- New parents may feel pressured to begin complementary foods early.

    - Messages from the media and baby food manufacturers
    - Advice from family and friends
    - Misinformed or misunderstood messages from the baby's caregiver
    - Misconceptions about frequency of feedings, milk production, richness of the mother's milk, sleep patterns, crying, and infant development

- Consequences of early introduction of complementary foods:

    - Frequent digestive upsets
    - Increased upper respiratory infections
    - Poor nutrient absorption
    - Excessive weight gain and risk of lifelong obesity
    - Early weaning

- How to introduce complementary foods:

    - Introduce a single-ingredient food one at a time at weekly intervals.

        - The baby's digestive system gets used to each new food.
        - The mother can identify food sensitivity.
        - It averts development of food intolerance or allergies.

- Introduce it at a time the baby will accept it.

  ‣ Initiate when the baby is still hungry after breastfeeding.
  ‣ If the baby objects to a particular food, withhold it for several weeks and offer it again.
  ‣ Avoid starting new foods when the baby is ill or recently had an inoculation.

- Allow breastfeeding to diminish slowly as other foods become the baby's primary nutrition.

  ‣ Breastmilk meets 75% of the baby's nutrient needs to 12 months of age.
  ‣ By 7 to 9 months, give one or two complementary feeds per day.
  ‣ By 9 to 12 months, give three family meals per day.
  ‣ Breastmilk continues to be nutritionally valuable into the second year.

> **Foods to avoid in the first year:**
> ► Cow's milk and milk products
> ► Citrus fruits and fruit juices
> ► Eggs
> ► Tomatoes
> ► Chocolate
> ► Fish
> ► Pork
> ► Peanuts and other nuts
> ► Wheat

- Types of complementary foods to give to the baby:

  - Introduce a texture compatible with the baby's ability to chew and swallow.
  - Go progressively from highly puréed food to food diluted with liquid, to texture that is coarser and then chunky, to finger foods, and then to table food.
  - Begin with about 1 teaspoon of creamy consistency and work up to a few tablespoons as determined by the baby's appetite.
  - Begin with foods high in protein, such as single-grain infant cereals, which provide additional energy and iron. Mix cereal with expressed milk or warm water.
  - Cereal is typically followed by vegetables, fruits, and meats in that order.
  - Babies do not require juice, desserts, or sweeteners.
  - Additional water will help rid the baby's body of waste products in solid foods.
  - In the second year of life, the child can share family meals.

    ‣ Prepare without excessive salt or spices.
    ‣ Cut into appropriate-sized pieces.
    ‣ Serve at moderate temperature.
    ‣ Vegetarian diets are inadequate for infants.

Signs of food intolerance:

▶ Runny nose, stuffiness, and constant cold-type symptoms

▶ Skin rashes, eczema, hives, and sore bottom

▶ Asthma

▶ Ear infections

▶ Intestinal upset, gas, diarrhea, spitting, and vomiting

▶ Fussiness, irritability, and coliclike behavior

▶ Poor weight gain due to malabsorption of food

▶ Red itchy eyes, swollen eyelids, dark circles under the eyes, constant tearing, and gelatin-like fluid in the eyes

Allergy Considerations

- Children with a family history of allergy need the prolonged protection that human milk provides.

  - They have increased susceptibility to ingested food proteins.
  - Avoiding potent allergenic foods during the first year reduces allergic reactions.

- Response ranges from sudden and clear-cut allergic reactions to slight fussiness or irritability.
- What mothers can do to reduce allergy symptoms:

  - Contact a caregiver to identify the allergen, and obtain medication to relieve symptoms.
  - Limit consumption of milk and eggs, especially during the last month of pregnancy.
  - Eat a variety of foods in moderation.
  - Exclude the offending food from the mother's diet.
  - If eliminating a food high in protein and calcium, substitute another food or supplement.
  - When beginning complementary foods, introduce one food at a time and wait 1 week for a possible reaction.
  - Limit exposure to other allergens.

    - Keep the baby's room free of dust and mold.
    - Keep the home free of dogs, cats, birds, and other pets for 6 months.
    - Keep the baby's skin free from contact with wool and lanolin products.
    - Avoid smoking near the baby and preferably nowhere in the home.

Weaning

Baby-Led Weaning

- This is the preferred method for weaning.
- The mother responds to feeding behavior and does not initiate feedings at other times.
- The baby drops feedings gradually.
- It occurs between periods of greatest developmental activity: 12 to 14 months, 18 months, 2 years, and 3 years.
- Signs a baby may be ready to wean:

  - The baby acts more self-reliant and goes for long stretches without nursing.
  - The baby accepts a drink or snack as a substitute.
  - The baby is easily distracted at the breast.
  - The baby spends less time at feedings.
  - The baby frequently refuses the breast.
  - The baby shows a greater interest in solid foods.

Mother-Led Weaning

- The mother attempts to end breastfeeding without cues from the baby.

  - She is impatient for the baby to wean and resents breastfeeding.
  - She feels pressure from others.
  - She received poor information or advice.
  - She plans to return to work.
  - She senses that her baby is no longer satisfied with breastfeeding.
  - She no longer enjoys breastfeeding.

- Adopt a nonjudgmental attitude, support the decision, and educate the mother about gradual weaning.

  - Eliminate the least preferred feeding first.
  - Allow at least 2 days for the baby and breasts to adjust.
  - Substitute a drink, snack, cuddling, or favorite activity.
  - Drop another feeding and continue gradually over several weeks or months.

Miscues that cause mothers to consider weaning:

▶ Crying is stressful and causes the mother to doubt that she is satisfying her baby's hunger.

▶ Teething, biting, or illness causes frustration or fatigue.

▶ Nighttime feeds and wakefulness are fatiguing to the mother.

▶ The mother believes weaning would simplify a family move, job change, illness, emotional upset, or other stressful situation.

▶ The mother wants to resume taking oral contraceptives.

SUPPORTING EXTENDED BREASTFEEDING

- ▪ The child may continue a preferred feeding and decrease frequency until weaning entirely.

- Minimal breastfeeding offers a compromise to total weaning.

  - ▪ Breastfeed one to three times a day.
  - ▪ Give complementary foods for remaining nourishment.

Emergency Weaning

- Drop every other feeding on the first day.
- Express just enough milk to relieve discomfort.
- Eliminate the remainder of the feedings.
- Include extra nurturing and attention for baby.
- Reduce breast swelling and pain with cabbage leaves or ice wrapped in a towel.
- Ibuprofen will help relieve pain.

Unintentional or Unplanned Early Weaning

- The mother starts giving occasional bottles and milk production diminishes.
- The mother contracts a serious illness or requires treatment that is contraindicated.
- The mother finds it difficult to combine work or school with breastfeeding.
- The baby suddenly refuses the breast and fails to resume breastfeeding.
- The mother becomes pregnant and has a history of miscarriage or premature birth.
- The mother has sore nipples because of pregnancy.

After Weaning

- Eliminating extra calories in the mother's diet can help avoid weight gain.
- Menstrual cycles may be irregular for a few months.
- The breasts may become soft, flat, or droopy for a few months.
- Stretch marks may be apparent on the breasts.
- Milk secretion may continue for several months. If spontaneous milk secretion continues up to 6 months, evaluate circumstances that may be stimulating milk production.

Tutorial for Students and Interns

Key Clinical Competencies

From *Clinical Competencies for IBCLC Practice* available at www.iblce.org.

- Assist mothers with overproduction of milk.
- Assist mothers with infants with food intolerances.

- Assist mothers with teething and biting.
- Assist mothers with toddler nursing.
- Assist mothers with nursing through pregnancy.
- Assist mothers with tandem nursing.
- Assist mothers with nursing strike or early baby-led weaning.
- Assist mothers with weaning issues.

Applying Theory to Practice

Consider what you would investigate and how you would respond to these statements by a mother. What would be your first statement to her?

1. The mother of a 2-day-old infant tells you he keeps turning his head when she tries to put him to breast.
2. A mother is home with her 5-day-old infant who is nursing every 1½ hours and is very fussy between feedings. She gave him 6 ounces of formula at the last feeding and he slept for 5 hours. She feels she may not have enough milk.
3. A mother of a 9-day-old baby is worried that her milk production is low. Her baby has been fussy and wanting to feed every 1½ hours for the past 24 hours and she is exhausted.
4. A mother is concerned that her 2-week-old baby falls asleep after one breast and does not feed on the other breast.
5. A mother fed her first two children formula. She is breastfeeding her 3-week-old infant and says he seems hungry all the time. She is reluctant to feed him more often than every 4 hours.
6. A mother tells you she is pleased that her 3-week-old baby is so easy to take care of. He sleeps all the time and hardly ever cries.
7. The mother of a 1-month-old baby tells you he shows a preference for her left breast, and she asks for help getting him to take the right breast.
8. A mother tells you her 1-month-old baby breastfed erratically for the past 2 days, as often as every 2 hours. He also is sleeping for longer stretches during the day. She asks what she is doing wrong.
9. A mother of a 1-month-old baby plans to attend a family gathering and will be staying with relatives for 2 days. She has never fed her baby in front of others and is worried about getting enough privacy for feedings.
10. A mother tells you she wants to wean her baby at 1 month of age.
11. A 6-week-old baby has a bad head cold. He cries constantly and is refusing to breastfeed. The mother sounds exhausted and discouraged.
12. The mother of a 2-month-old infant wants to supplement him with expressed breastmilk after every feeding because he is such a big baby and she thinks he needs more than he gets at a breastfeeding.
13. A mother tells you she was approached at a shopping mall when she was breastfeeding her 3-month-old baby and was asked to go to a more private place.

14. A mother is diagnosed with Crohn's disease when her exclusively breastfed daughter is 3 months old. She was told she must stop breastfeeding because of the medication she needs for her disease.

15. A mother asks you when her baby will start sleeping for longer periods at night. She is still waking every 3 hours to nurse at 3 months of age.

16. A relative suggested to the mother of a 4-month-old exclusively breastfed baby that she is overfeeding him.

17. A mother just returned from her baby's 4-month visit to the pediatrician. She was told to start complementary foods because her baby seems hungry all the time. She thought she was supposed to wait until 6 months to begin complementary foods.

18. A mother is concerned because her 5-month-old baby stays on each breast for only a few brief minutes at every feeding. She worries that he is losing interest in breastfeeding or may not be getting enough to eat. She asks if she should start supplemental feedings.

19. A mother tells you her 6-month-old baby has suddenly stopped breastfeeding.

20. A mother tells you her 7-month-old baby has started biting her during feedings. She had wanted to breastfeed until at least 1 year.

21. A mother reacted sharply to her 8-month-old baby when he bit her during a feeding. Now he refuses to breastfeed, and the mother feels responsible.

22. A mother tells you she is exhausted because her 8-month-old baby refuses to be with anyone but her and wants to be held all the time.

23. A mother tells you her 9-month-old baby suddenly started nursing more frequently than before. She wonders if it is due to a decrease in her milk supply.

24. The mother of a 1-year-old baby tells you that her baby wants to nurse whenever she gets involved in doing something. She is getting frustrated because she can never seem to accomplish anything.

25. The father of a 12-month-old baby is pressuring his wife to wean their baby. She wants to continue.

26. A mother asks how she should coordinate breastfeeding with complementary foods when she starts them at 6 months.

27. The mother of a 14-month-old baby worries that her baby reacted to something she ate because he suddenly has a rash on his face.

28. A woman in your prenatal breastfeeding class tells you that she is still breastfeeding her 14-month-old baby and doesn't want to wean. But she worries about how she can manage breastfeeding both babies after she delivers the new baby.

29. The mother of an 18-month-old toddler tells you that her daughter embarrasses her when they are in public by insisting on nursing and becoming disruptive when the mother attempts to distract her.

30. A mother tells you she wanted to let her baby decide when to wean but he is 20 months old and hasn't shown any signs of wanting to stop breastfeeding. She asks what she can do to start weaning.

31. A mother asks if it is safe for her to sleep with her infant.
32. Four months after her 1-year-old baby weaned, a mother continues to leak milk and asks how long it will last.
33. A woman in your prenatal breastfeeding class says when she was on an airplane recently there was a baby who cried during most of the flight. She is worried that she will have the same problem.

Appendix A
Seeking Employment as an International Board Certified Lactation Consultant (IBCLC)

Judith Lauwers, BA, IBCLC

Before seeking employment as an IBCLC, you will want to prepare for the initial contact. If you are applying for an existing position that is vacant, you may be competing with several qualified individuals and will need to stand out from among them. Plan to complete an application and submit a current résumé and cover letter highlighting your potential contributions as an IBCLC. If you are proposing the creation of a new position, you can illustrate the value of an IBCLC and present yourself as the best candidate for such a position. In addition to writing a current résumé and a cover letter that highlights the role you can play as an IBCLC, preparation will include writing a draft of your job proposal.

Résumé

A well-written résumé is essential when applying to a facility for employment. If you already have one, make sure it is up to date and includes all employment and other experience. A résumé should showcase your talents and describe your background and work experience. Limit it to one page, as employers tend to only look at the first page if there are more pages. If this is your first résumé, you may want to contact a résumé service, which you can locate through the Web. Simply search using the words *resume* and *write* to find several sites. Be prepared to submit a curriculum vitae (CV) if requested. A CV lists all of your academic achievements, professional memberships, publications, and other scholarly accomplishments. It is usually much lengthier than a résumé and is more than a potential employer may want to read. You can note at the bottom of your résumé that a curriculum vitae is available upon request.

Proposing a New Position

First, try to establish a base of support with colleagues who will champion your cause. Learn what the staff want or need in terms of breastfeeding assistance. Document the need for lactation services with statistics of breastfeeding rates and mothers and babies who experienced problems. Comparing breastfeeding rates with those of a competing hospital that employs an IBCLC will strengthen your case, demonstrating how an IBCLC position would benefit the hospital. Compile a brief bibliography of documents on why and when women stop breastfeeding. In the United States, you can include the *Healthy People 2010* goals and statements from the American Academy of Pediatrics and the Academy of Breastfeeding Medicine. Also cite ILCA's *Clinical Guidelines for the Establishment of Exclusive Breastfeeding.*

For proposing a new position, identify someone who knows the power structure at the facility. Most often this would be the manager of the mother–baby unit. Begin your cover letter by explaining the role of an IBCLC in the healthcare team and the value to families. You can enclose brochures from ILCA and from the International Board of Lactation Consultant Examiners to supplement your description. Provide rationale for the facility to hire an IBCLC, and explain how the facility would benefit. Briefly describe how you see yourself functioning in the facility, highlighting some of the responsibilities listed under *Elements of an IBCLC Job Description* below. Include the potential cost to the facility for your services and how those costs could be offset.

You can postpone submitting a formal proposal until you have had an interview to determine the facility's interest and what they would look for in a position. Be prepared with a draft that outlines the specific role you propose so that you can suggest options. You may even want to include the list of options with your cover letter to illustrate the varied scope of an IBCLC practice. If you do this, be sure to indicate that one person cannot accomplish everything on the list! Present it as a list of potential tasks from which to design a job description.

Applying for an Existing Position

If you are applying for an existing position, you can begin by learning as much as possible about the current position. If you can obtain a copy of the existing job description, you can highlight the areas where you can benefit the facility. Enclosing brochures from ILCA and from the International Board of Lactation Consultant Examiners will demonstrate your professionalism and help you to stand out among the other candidates. In your cover letter, briefly describe how you see yourself functioning in the facility. Suggest any new responsibilities listed under *Elements of an IBCLC Job Description* that are not already in the current job description. Be prepared with a draft of a new job description that outlines the specific role you propose so that you can suggest options.

Submitting the Proposal

Most facilities begin the hiring process for an existing position in their human resources department. Increasingly, applications are submitted online via a Web site. If you do this, follow up with a letter and résumé to the manager of the mother–baby unit. State the position you seek and why you are applying to the particular facility. Explain that you submitted an application online to the human resources department, express your interest in a personal interview, and invite the manager to contact you with any questions. Send a copy of these materials to the human resources department as well. Indicate that you submitted an application online and wanted to make sure they received it. This is an important step, since you cannot be sure that the online application arrived. If you complete an application in person, you will still want to follow up with a mailing to the manager of the mother–baby unit.

Elements of an IBCLC Job Description

IBCLC job descriptions vary depending on the facility's needs. Job responsibilities often evolve to reflect the personality and interests of the person holding the position. If a position already exists, you can review the current job description and highlight where your background and talents seem tailor-made for their position. When proposing a new position, determine how an IBCLC can best fit into the facility, and edit the job proposal accordingly. A job description needs to reflect what would be most appropriate for the particular practice setting.

The job proposal may include the expertise required, the services provided, the resources needed for the position, and ways to cover the cost of the position. You can select from among the items below to construct your personalized job proposal. When you are employed, you can continue to tweak it to reflect your personality and talents.

Professional Requirements of the IBCLC

- IBLCE certification
- Specialized training in lactation
- Membership in a professional association
- Graduation from an accredited school, if applicable
- Current licensure in state, if applicable
- Skills, knowledge, and interest in promoting breastfeeding
- Communication skills essential for interactions with patients, families, colleagues
- Knowledge of cultural, psychological, psychosocial, nutritional, and pharmacological aspects of breastfeeding
- Understanding of current breastfeeding practices and research findings
- Regular continuing education through seminars, workshops, and professional networking
- Experience in the type of work setting
- Support of work-setting philosophy and policies
- Understanding of adult learning principles
- Ability to provide leadership for activities to promote breastfeeding in the community

Objectives of Employing an IBCLC

- Increase revenue through an increased number of clients choosing the facility because of customer satisfaction with enhanced services.
- Enhance employer's reputation as a concerned provider of health care to mothers and babies.
- Achieve better health for babies and mothers.
- Provide consistent breastfeeding teaching and support.
- Increase the percentage of mothers choosing to breastfeed.

- Increase the percentage of mothers continuing to breastfeed exclusively until 6 months and with appropriate complementary foods to at least 1 year
- Increase customer satisfaction, and provide positive breastfeeding experiences for mothers and babies

Teaching Services

- Prenatal breastfeeding classes
- In-hospital breastfeeding classes
- Postpartum classes after babies are home
- In-service education for staff
- Orientation of staff
- Maintaining a resource center for patient and staff educational materials
- Teaching of staff through a mentorship or preceptor program

Services to Mothers

- Develop, implement, and evaluate breastfeeding programs for patient and family education both prenatally and postpartum.
- Purchase, review, and evaluate breastfeeding audiovisual materials and other parent teaching aids.
- Provide breastfeeding assessment, support, and counseling to both inpatients and outpatients.

  - Conduct daily rounds of breastfeeding mothers.
  - Revisit mothers who are experiencing problems.
  - Perform physical breastfeeding assessments.
  - Develop plans of care with mothers.
  - Provide problem-solving advice and support.
  - Provide anticipatory guidance.
  - Document teaching and progress on patient's charts.

- Coordinate or provide home follow-up through phone calls, postcards, or visits.
- Offer a 24-hour answering machine, hot line, or warm line.
- Make appropriate referrals to physicians, breastfeeding support groups, and other services.
- Coordinate mothers providing breastmilk for a donor milk bank
- Coordinate, instruct, and follow up with mothers using breastfeeding aids.
- Provide a drop-in clinic to weigh infants, discuss problems, and give anticipatory guidance to mothers and families.

Working with the Healthcare Team

- Collaborate on the development, implementation, and evaluation of teaching aids.
- Consult with physicians and nursing staff on breastfeeding protocols and standards of care.
- Review and maintain a file of current research and literature.
- Disseminate current information and research data on breastfeeding.
- Serve as a resource for parents, staff, physicians, students, and volunteer support group counselors.
- Initiate case conferences, and confer with staff on patient needs.
- Discuss appropriate referrals with primary care providers.
- Provide an on-call service for consultations with staff.
- Collaborate as a team member with staff and physicians to provide comprehensive care.
- Participate in interdisciplinary documentation by charting assessments, interventions, and results.
- Confer with nursing personnel on family progress, special needs, and continuity of care.
- Provide consultation to other facilities on a shared service basis.
- Provide input for the creation or revision of hospital polices affecting breastfeeding.
- Provide leadership on breastfeeding committees.

Writing, Reviewing, and Revising Printed Materials

- Establish, review, and revise policies, procedures, and standards of care that affect breastfeeding.
- Develop, review, and revise breastfeeding policies, care plans, and patient literature.
- Develop and revise a charting system for documentation, teaching, and progress notes.
- Maintain statistics to assess the effectiveness of IBCLC services.
- Prepare a monthly breastfeeding newsletter.

Equipment and Other Resources Needed

- Office space with a sink and large enough for a stroller and the mother's support person
- Desk and chair
- Computer with Internet access
- File cabinets
- Telephone
- Answering machine or voice mail

- Beeper
- Comfortable cushioned armchair with footstool for mothers
- Additional chairs (for fathers, grandparents, lactation consultant)
- Bed or couch to teach side-lying position
- Positioning aids (nursing pillows, etc.)
- Electric breast pumps and other devices
- Baby scale
- Secretarial help
- System for tracking and billing pumps if rentals will be part of the service
- Retail space with inventory of items for purchase
- System for handling stock, reordering, and finances
- Funds for texts and continuing education

Covering the Fee for the Services of an IBCLC

- Limited amount of inpatient teaching and rounds included in the OB care package, with additional more complex intervention or problem solving for a fee (capitation contract needs to highlight this as a "value added" service and include the costs).
- Use of (and charging for) clinically indicated lactation-related supplies.
- A prenatal class.
- After discharge follow-up: telephone counseling, office visit, home visit.

Appendix B
International Lactation Consultant Association
*Standards of Practice for International Board Certified
Lactation Consultants*
Approved by the Board of Directors October, 2005.

Preface
This is the third edition of *Standards of Practice for International Board Certified
Lactation Consultants (IBCLCs)* published by the International Lactation
Consultant Association (ILCA). All individuals practicing as a currently certi-
fied IBCLC should adhere to ILCA's standards of practice and the International
Board of Lactation Consultant Examiners (IBLCE) *Code of Ethics for International
Board Certified Lactation Consultants* in all interactions with clients, families, and
other healthcare professionals. ILCA recognizes the certification conferred by
the IBLCE as the worldwide professional credential for lactation consultants.

Quality practice and service are the core responsibilities of a profession to
the public. Standards of practice are stated measures or levels of quality that are
models for the conduct and evaluation of practice.

Standards of Practice

- promote consistency by encouraging a common systematic approach.
- are sufficiently specific in content to guide daily practice.
- provide a recommended framework for the development of policies and protocols, educational programs, and quality improvement efforts.
- Standards are intended for use in diverse practice settings and cultural contexts.

Standard 1. Professional Responsibilities
The IBCLC has a responsibility to maintain professional conduct and to practice
in an ethical manner, accountable for professional actions and legal responsibilities.

1.1   Adhere to these ILCA Standards of Practice and the IBLCE Code of Ethics.
1.2   Practice within the scope of the International Code of Marketing of Breast-
      milk Substitutes and all subsequent World Health Association resolutions.
1.3   Maintain an awareness of conflict of interest in all aspects of work, espe-
      cially when profiting from the rental or sale of breastfeeding equipment
      and services.
1.4   Act as an advocate for breastfeeding women, infants, and children.
1.5   Assist the mother in maintaining a breastfeeding relationship with her child.
1.6   Maintain and expand knowledge and skills for lactation consultant practice
      by participating in continuing education.

1.7 Undertake periodic and systematic evaluation of one's clinical practice.
1.8 Support and promote well-designed research in human lactation and breast-feeding, and base clinical practice, whenever possible, on such research.

Standard 2. Legal Considerations

The IBCLC is obligated to practice within the laws of the geopolitical region and setting in which she/he works. The IBCLC must practice with consideration for rights of privacy and with respect for matters of a confidential nature.

2.1 Work within the policies and procedures of the institution where employed, or if self-employed, have identifiable policies and procedures to follow.
2.2 Clearly state applicable fees prior to providing care.
2.3 Obtain informed consent from all clients prior to:

- assessing or intervening
- reporting relevant information to other healthcare professional(s)
- taking photographs for any purpose
- seeking publication of information associated with the consultation

2.4 Protect client confidentiality at all times.
2.5 Maintain records according to legal and ethical practices within the work setting.

Standard 3. Clinical Practice

The clinical practice of the IBCLC focuses on providing clinical lactation care and management. This is best accomplished by promoting optimal health, through collaboration and problem- solving with the client and other members of the health care team. The role of the IBCLC includes:

- assessment, planning, intervention, and evaluation of care in a variety of situations
- anticipatory guidance and prevention of problems
- complete, accurate, and timely documentation of care
- communication and collaboration with other health care professionals

3.1 Assessment

    3.1.1 Obtain and document an appropriate history of the breastfeeding mother and child.
    3.1.2 Systematically collect objective and subjective information.
    3.1.3 Discuss with the mother and document as appropriate all assessment information.

3.2 Plan

    3.2.1 Analyze assessment information to identify issues and/or problems.
    3.2.2 Develop a plan of care based on identified issues.

3.2.3   Arrange for follow-up evaluation where indicated.

3.3   Implementation

3.3.1   Implement the plan of care in a manner appropriate to the situation and acceptable to the mother.

3.3.2   Utilize translators as needed.

3.3.3   Exercise principles of optimal health, safety, and universal precautions.

3.3.4   Provide appropriate oral and written instructions and/or demonstration of interventions, procedures, and techniques.

3.3.5   Facilitate referral to other health care professionals, community services, and support groups as needed.

3.3.6   Use equipment appropriately:

- refrain from unnecessary or excessive use.
- assure cleanliness and good operating condition.
- discuss the risks and benefits of recommended equipment including financial considerations.
- demonstrate the correct use and care of equipment.
- evaluate safety and effectiveness of use.

3.3.7   Document and communicate to health care providers as appropriate:

- assessment information
- suggested interventions
- instructions provided
- evaluations of outcomes
- modifications of the plan of care
- follow-up strategies

3.4   Evaluation

3.4.1   Evaluate outcomes of planned interventions.

3.4.2   Modify the care plan based on the evaluation of outcomes.

Standard 4. Breastfeeding Education and Counseling

Breastfeeding education and counseling are integral parts of the care provided by the IBCLC.

4.1   Educate parents and families to encourage informed decision-making about infant and child feeding.

4.2   Utilize a pragmatic problem-solving approach, sensitive to the learner's culture, questions, and concerns.

4.3   Provide anticipatory guidance (teaching) to:

- promote optimal breastfeeding practices.
- minimize the potential for breastfeeding problems or complications.

4.4   Provide positive feedback and emotional support for continued breastfeeding, especially in difficult or complicated circumstances.

4.5   Share current evidence-based information and clinical skills in collaboration with other health care providers.

Source: International Lactation Consultant Association

Appendix C
Code of Ethics for International Board of Certified Lactation Consultants

International Board of Lactation Consultant Manager.
Effective December 1, 2004.

Preamble

It is in the best interests of the profession of lactation consultants and the public it serves that there be a Code of Ethics to provide guidance to lactation consultants in their professional practice and conduct. These ethical principles guide the profession and outline commitments and obligations of the lactation consultant to self, client, colleagues, society, and the profession.

The purpose of the International Board of Lactation Consultant Examiners (IBLCE) is to assist in the protection of the health, safety, and welfare of the public by establishing and enforcing qualifications of certification and for issuing voluntary credentials to individuals who have attained those qualifications. The IBLCE has adopted this Code to apply to all individuals who hold the credential of International Board Certified Lactation Consultant (IBCLC), Registered Lactation Consultant.

Principles of Ethical Practice

The International Board Certified Lactation Consultant, Registered Lactation Consultant, shall act in a manner that safeguards the interests of individual clients, justifies public trust in her/his competence, and enhances the reputation of the profession. The International Board Certified Lactation Consultant, Registered Lactation Consultant, is personally accountable for his/her practice and, in the exercise of professional accountability, must:

1. Provide professional services with objectivity and with respect for the unique needs and values of individuals.
2. Avoid discrimination against other individuals on the basis of race, creed, religion, gender, sexual orientation, age, and national origin.
3. Fulfill professional commitments in good faith.
4. Conduct herself/ himself with honesty, integrity, and fairness.
5. Remain free of conflict of interest while fulfilling the objectives and maintaining the integrity of the lactation consultant profession.
6. Maintain confidentiality.
7. Base her/his practice on scientific principles, current research, and information.
8. Take responsibility and accept accountability for personal competence in practice.
9. Recognize and exercise professional judgment within the limits of her/his qualifications. This principle includes seeking counsel and making referrals to appropriate providers.
10. Inform the public and colleagues of his/her services by using factual information. An International Board Certified Lactation Consultant, Registered Lactation Consultant, will not advertise in a false or misleading manner.

11. Provide sufficient information to enable clients to make informed decisions.
12. Provide information about appropriate products in a manner that is neither false nor misleading.
13. Permit use of her/his name for the purpose of certifying that lactation consultant services have been rendered only if she/he provided those services.
14. Present professional qualifications and credentials accurately, using IBCLC, RLC, only when certification is current and authorized by the IBLCE, and complying with all requirements when seeking initial or continued certification from the IBLCE. The lactation consultant is subject to disciplinary action for aiding another person in violating any IBLCE requirements or aiding another person in representing himself/herself as an IBCLC, RLC when he/she is not.
15. Report to an appropriate person or authority when it appears that the health or safety of colleagues is at risk, as such circumstances may compromise standards of practice and care.
16. Refuse any gift, favor, or hospitality from patients or clients currently in her/his care which might be interpreted as seeking to exert influence to obtain preferential consideration.
17. Disclose any financial or other conflicts of interest in relevant organizations providing goods or services. Ensure that professional judgment is not influenced by any commercial considerations.
18. Present substantiated information, and interpret controversial information without personal bias, recognizing that legitimate differences of opinion exist.
19. Withdraw voluntarily from professional practice if the lactation consultant has engaged in any substance abuse that could affect his/her practice; has been adjudged by a court to be mentally incompetent; or has a physical, emotional or mental disability that affects her/his practice in a manner that could harm the client.
20. Obtain maternal consent to photograph, audiotape, or videotape a mother and/or her infant(s) for educational or professional purposes.
21. Submit to disciplinary action under the following circumstance: If convicted of a crime under the laws of the practitioner's country which is a felony or a misdemeanor, an essential element of which is dishonesty, and which is related to the practice of lactation consulting; if disciplined by a state, province, or other local government and at least one of the grounds for the discipline is the same or substantially equivalent to these principles; if committed an act of misfeasance or malfeasance which is directly related to the practice of the profession as determined by a court of competent jurisdiction, a licensing board, or an agency of a governmental body; or if violated a Principle set forth in the Code of Ethics for International Board Certified Lactation Consultants which was in force at the time of the violation.
22. Accept the obligation to protect society and the profession by upholding the Code of Ethics for International Board Certified Lactation Consultants and by reporting alleged violations of the Code through the defined review process of the IBLCE.

23. Require and obtain consent to share clinical concerns and information with the physician or other primary health care provider before initiating a consultation.
24. IBCLC, RLCs must adhere to those provisions of the International Code of Marketing of Breast-Milk Substitutes and subsequent resolutions which pertain to health workers.
25. Understand, recognize, respect, and acknowledge intellectual property rights, including but not limited to copyrights (which apply to written material, photographs, slides, illustrations, etc.), trademarks, service marks, and patents.

Source: International Board of Lactation Consultant Examiners

Appendix D
Summary of the International Code of Marketing of Breastmilk Substitutes

Code Provision	Implications to Consider
Under the scope of the Code, items marketed or otherwise represented to be suitable as human milk substitutes can include foods and beverages such as: • Infant Formula • Other milk products • Cereals • Vegetable, fruit and other pureed preparations • Juices and baby teas • Follow-on milks • Bottled water	Whether or not a product is considered to be within this definition will depend on how it is promoted for infants. Any products that are marketed or represented as suitable substitutes to human milk will fall into this category. Since babies should receive only human milk for the first six months, any other food or drink promoted for use during this time will be a human milk substitute.
Regarding advertising and information, the Code recommends that: • Advertising of human milk substitutes, bottles, and teats to the public not be permitted • Educational materials explain the benefits of breastfeeding, the health hazards associated with bottle feeding, the costs of using infant formula, and the difficulty of reversing the decision not to breastfeed. • Product labels clearly state the superiority of breastfeeding, the need for the advice of a healthcare worker, and a warning about health hazards; and they show no pictures of babies, or other pictures or text idealizing the use of infant formula	Health workers such as lactation consultants and breastfeeding counselors need to press their legislators for measures that will implement the Code in full. This would protect mothers from advertising in parent magazines and on television. It would also prevent direct company contact with mothers through hot lines, Internet sites, mailings, home-delivered supplies of formula, and baby clubs.

Code Provision	Implications to Consider
Regarding samples and supplies, the Code recommends that: • No free samples be given to pregnant women, mothers, or their families • No free or low-cost supplies of human milk substitutes be given to maternity wards, hospitals, or any other part of the healthcare system	Under the Code, free or low-cost supplies can be distributed only outside of the healthcare system and must be continued for as long as the infant needs them. In the United States, this is usually one year. Elsewhere, it is for at least six months. The healthcare system encompasses healthcare workers, including lactation consultants and breastfeeding counselors.
Regarding healthcare facilities and healthcare workers, the Code recommends that: • There be no product displays, posters, or distribution or promotional materials • No gifts or samples be given to healthcare workers • Product information for health professionals be limited to what is factual and scientific.	This provision also covers bottles that are provided and shown in advertisements by breast pump companies that are clearly feeding bottles, even when no teats are shown. Pens and pads of paper with the name of a formula company are examples of gifts.

Appendix E
Ten Steps To Successful Breastfeeding:
Self-Appraisal Tool

Step 1. Have a written breastfeeding policy that is routinely communicated to all health care staff.

1.1   Does the health facility have an explicit written policy for protecting, promoting, and supporting breastfeeding that addresses all Ten Steps to Successful Breastfeeding in maternity services?
1.2   Does the policy protect breastfeeding by prohibiting all promotion of and group instruction for using breastmilk substitutes, feeding bottles, and teats?
1.3   Is the breastfeeding policy available so all staff who take care of mothers and babies can refer to it?
1.4   Is the breastfeeding policy posted or displayed in all areas of the health facility that serve mothers, infants, and/or children?
1.5   Is there a mechanism for evaluating the effectiveness of the policy?

Step 2. Train all healthcare staff in skills necessary to implement this policy.

2.1   Are all staff aware of the advantages of breastfeeding and acquainted with the facility's policy and services to protect, promote, and support breastfeeding?
2.2   Are all staff caring for women and infants oriented to the breastfeeding policy on the hospital on their arrival?
2.3   Is training on breastfeeding and lactation management given to all staff caring for women and infants within 6 months of their arrival?
2.4   Does the training cover at least eight of the Ten Steps?
2.5   Is the training on breastfeeding and lactation management at least 18 hours in total, including a minimum of 3 hours of supervised clinical experience?
2.6   Has the health care facility arranged for specialized training in lactation management of specific staff members?

Step 3. Inform all pregnant women about the benefits and management of breastfeeding.

3.1   Does the hospital include an antenatal care clinic or an antenatal inpatient ward?
3.2   If yes, are most pregnant women attending these antenatal services informed about the benefits and management of breastfeeding?

3.3   Do antenatal records indicate whether breastfeeding has been discussed with the pregnant woman?

3.4   Is a mother's antenatal record available at the time of delivery?

3.5   Are pregnant women protected from oral or written promotion of and group instruction for artificial feeding?

3.6   Does the health care facility take into account a woman's intention to breastfeed when deciding on the use of a sedative, an analgesic, or an anaesthetic (if any) during labor and delivery?

3.7   Are staff familiar with the effects of such medicaments on breastfeeding?

3.8   Does a woman who has never breastfed or who has previously encountered problems with breastfeeding receive special attention and support from the staff of the healthcare facility?

Step 4. Help mothers initiate breastfeeding within a half-hour of birth.

4.1   Are mothers whose deliveries are normal given their babies to hold, with skin contact, within a half-hour of completion of the second stage of labor and allowed to remain with them for at least the first hour?

4.2   Are the mothers offered help by a staff member to initiate breastfeeding during this first hour?

4.3   Are mothers who have had caesarean deliveries given their babies to hold, with skin contact, within a half-hour after they are able to respond to their babies?

4.4   Do the babies born by caesarean delivery stay with their mothers with skin contact at this time, for at least 30 minutes?

Step 5. Show mothers how to breastfeed and how to maintain lactation, even if they should be separated from their infants.

5.1   Does nursing staff offer all mothers further assistance with breastfeeding within 6 hours of delivery?

5.2   Are most breastfeeding mothers able to demonstrate how to position and attach their baby correctly for breastfeeding?

5.3   Are breastfeeding mothers shown how to express their milk or given information on expression or advised of where they can get help, should they need it?

5.4   Are staff members or counselors who have specialized training in breastfeeding and lactation management available full-time to advise mothers during their stay in healthcare facilities and in preparation for discharge?

5.5   Does a woman who has never breastfed or who has previously encountered problems with breastfeeding receive special attention and support from the staff of the healthcare facility?

5.6 Are mothers of babies in special care helped to establish and maintain lactation by frequent expression of milk?

Step 6. Give newborn infants no food or drink other than breastmilk, unless medically indicated.

6.1 Do staff have a clear understanding of what the few acceptable reasons are for prescribing food or drink other than breastmilk for breastfeeding babies?
6.2 Do breastfeeding babies receive no other food or drink (other than breastmilk) unless medically indicated?
6.3 Are any breastmilk substitutes including special formulas that are used in the facility purchased in the same way as any other foods or medicines?
6.4 Do the health facility and all healthcare workers refuse free or low-cost supplies of breastmilk substitutes, paying close to retail market price for any? (Low-cost = below 80% open-market retail cost. Breastmilk substitutes intended for experimental use or "professional evaluation" should also be purchased at 80% or more of retail price.)
6.5 Is all promotion for infant foods or drinks other than breastmilk absent from the facility?

Step 7. Practice rooming-in—allow mothers and infants to remain together—24 hours a day.

7.1 Do mothers and infants remain together (rooming-in 24 hours a day), except for periods of up to an hour for hospital procedures or if separation is medically indicated?
7.2 Does rooming-in start within an hour of a normal birth?
7.3 Does rooming-in start within an hour of when a caesarean mother can respond to her baby?

Step 8. Encourage breastfeeding on demand.

8.1 By placing no restrictions on the frequency or length of breastfeeding, do staff show that they are aware of the importance of breastfeeding on demand?
8.2 Are mothers advised to breastfeed their babies whenever their babies are hungry and as often as their babies want to breastfeed?

Step 9. Give no artificial teats or pacifiers (also called dummies or soothers) to breastfeeding infants.

9.1 Are babies who have started to breastfeed cared for without any bottle feeds?
9.2 Are babies who have started to breastfeed cared for without using pacifiers?

9.3   Do breastfeeding mothers learn that they should not give any bottles or pacifiers to their babies?

9.4   By accepting no free or low-cost feeding bottles, teats, or pacifiers, do the facility and the caregivers demonstrate that these should be avoided?

Step 10. Foster the establishment of breastfeeding support groups, and refer mothers to them on discharge from the hospital or clinic.

10.1 Does the hospital give education to key family members so that they can support the breastfeeding mother at home?

10.2 Are breastfeeding mothers referred to breastfeeding support groups, if any are available?

10.3 Does the hospital have a system of follow-up support for breastfeeding mothers after they are discharged, such as early postnatal or lactation clinic check-ups, home visits, telephone calls?

10.4 Does the facility encourage and facilitate the formation of mother-to-mother or health care worker-to-mother support groups?

10.5 Does the facility allow breastfeeding counseling by trained mother-to-mother support group counselors in its maternity services?

Used with permission of UNICEF/WHO.

Appendix F
Documentation Forms
Breastfeeding Descriptors for Documenting a Feeding

You may chart two types of feedings in one session. For example, a mother and baby may need considerable assistance with attachment. After the latch is achieved, the baby demonstrates nutritive sucking with audible swallows. This would be charted as *FBF → GBF.* Another example: You observe a baby that has some difficulty latching and the mom is poorly positioned. After offering assistance, the mother and baby overcome the obstacles and have an excellent feeding with lots of swallows. This would be charted as *Initial → PBF after assistance EBF.* Any rating below Excellent Breastfeed or Good Breastfeed will require further documentation that describes the problem and any help that is given.

Descriptor	Meaning	Elements observed
EBF	• Excellent breastfeed Note: It would be unusual to see an excellent breastfeed in the first 24 to 48 hours of life.	• Baby can latch on without difficulty • Sucks are nice and deep with a nice steady rhythm • Pauses are brief, and baby quickly resumes sucking again • Can hear baby swallowing frequently, sometimes with each suck • Mother does not need assistance positioning the baby or latching him on • No nipple discomfort
GBF	• Good breastfeed	• Baby can latch on without any difficulty • Sucks are nice and deep with a nice steady rhythm • Pauses are brief, and baby resumes sucking again without being moved or prodded • Some swallowing is heard • Mother requires a little help with positioning or latch-on • No nipple discomfort

Descriptor	Meaning	Elements observed
FBF	• Fair breastfeed	• Baby is able to latch on to the breast and once on is able to stay on • Sucks are short and quick; only occasionally may there be a nice deep suck; no steady rhythm • Mother has to stroke or prod infant to resume sucking • An occasional swallow may be heard, but usually no swallowing is heard • Mother requires a lot of assistance with positioning and latch-on • Mother could be experiencing nipple discomfort
PBF	• Poor breastfeed	• Roots for the breast, licks the nipple • Latches on, but has difficulty doing it • Once latched-on he does not stay on the breast or if he does he does not suck • No swallowing is heard • Mother requires a lot of assistance with positioning and latch-on • Mother could have nipple discomfort or pain
ABF	• Attempted breastfeed	• Roots and licks at the nipple • Unable to latch on to the nipple • Mother requires a great deal of assistance
OBF	• No breastfeed	• No effort at the breast (too sleepy, lethargic, no interest) • Pushes away from the breast, fights or cries, or both • Despite lots of assistance, unable to accomplish a feed

Printed by permission of Breastfeeding Support Consultants (Barger, Kutner, 1996).

UNICEF BREASTfeed Observation Form

B-R-E-A-S-T FEED OBSERVATION

Mother's name _____

Date_____

Infant's age _____

[Bracketed items refer only to the newborn infant, not to the older infant who sits up.]

Signs that breastfeeding is going well:	**Signs of possible difficulty:**
Body Position	
___ Mother relaxed and comfortable	___ Shoulders tense, leans over baby
___ Infant's body close to mother	___ Infant's body away from mother's
___ Infant's head and body straight	___ Infant must twist neck
___ Infant's chin touching breast	___ Infant's chin does not touch breast
___ [Infant's bottom supported]	___ [Only shoulder or head supported]
Responses	
___ Infant reaches for breast if hungry	___ No response to breast
___ [Infant roots for breast]	___ [No rooting observed]
___ Infant explores breast with tongue	___ Infant not interested in breast
___ Infant calm and alert at breast	___ Infant restless or fussy
___ Infant stays attached to breast	___ Infant slips off breast
___ Signs of milk ejection: [leaking, after pains]	___ No sign of milk ejection

Signs that breastfeeding is going well:	Signs of possible difficulty:
Emotional bonding	
___ Secure, confident hold	___ Nervous, shaking, or limp hold
___ Face-to-face attention from mother	___ No mother/infant eye contact
___ Much touching by mother	___ Little touching between mother and infant
Anatomy	
___ Breasts soft and full	___ Breasts engorged and hard
___ Nipples stick out, protractile	___ Nipples flat or inverted
___ Skin appears healthy	___ Fissures or redness of skin
___ Breast looks round during feed	___ Breast looks stretched or pulled
Suckling	
___ Mouth wide open	___ Mouth closed, points forward
___ Lower lip turned outward	___ Lower lip turned in
___ Tongue cupped around breast	___ Cannot see infant's tongue
___ Cheeks round	___ Cheeks tense or pulled in
___ Slow deep sucks, bursts with pauses	___ Rapid sucks
___ Can see or hear swallowing	___ Can hear smacking or clicking
Time spent suckling	
___ Infant releases breast	___ Mother takes infant off breast
Infant suckled for _____ minutes	

Notes:

From *Breastfeeding Management and Promotion in a Baby Friendly Hospital: An 18-Hour Course for Maternity Staff*, UNICEF/WHO, 1993.

The LATCH method

	0	1	2
L Latch	Too sleepy or reluctant No sustained latch or suck achieved	Repeated attempts for sustained latch or suck Hold nipple in mouth Stimulate to suck	Grasps breast Tongue down Lips flanged Rhythmical sucking
A Audible swallowing	None	A few with stimulation	Spontaneous and intermittent <24 hours old Spontaneous and frequent >24 hours old
T Type of nipple	Inverted	Flat	Everted (after stimulation)
C Comfort (breast/nipple)	Engorged Cracked, bleeding, large blisters, or bruises Severe discomfort	Filling Reddened/small blisters or bruises Mild/moderate discomfort	Soft Nontender
H Hold (positioning)	Full assist (staff holds infant at breast)	Minimal assist (i.e., elevate head of bed; place pillows for support) Teach one side; mother does other Staff holds and then mother takes over	No assist from staff Mother able to position and hold infant

Source: Jenson D, Wallace S, Kelsay P (1994). LATCH: A breastfeeding charting system and documentation tool. *JOGNN*, 23(1):29. Reprinted with permission of Lippincott-Raven Publishers and authors.

The Mother–Baby Assessment (MBA) Method

	M	B	HELP
Signaling	x	x	
Positioning	x	x	
Fixing	x		
Milk Transfer			
Ending			

Total Score 5 (With Help)

This is an assessment method for rating the progress of a mother and baby who are learning to breastfeed.

For every step, each person—both mother and baby—should receive an *x* before either one can be scored on the following step. If the observer does not observe any of the designated indicators, score 0 for that person on that step. If help is needed at any step for either the mother or the baby, check *Help* for that step. This notation will not change the total score for mother and baby.

1. Signaling

- Mother watches and listens for baby's cues. She may hold, stroke, rock, talk to baby. She stimulates baby if he is sleepy, calms baby if he is fussy.
- Baby gives readiness cues: stirring, alertness, rooting, sucking, hand-to-mouth, vocal cues, cry.

2. Positioning

- Mother holds baby in good alignment within latch-on range of nipple. Baby's body is slightly flexed, entire ventral surface facing mother's body. Baby's head and shoulders are supported.
- Baby roots well at breast, opens mouth wide, tongue cupped and covering lower gum.

3. Fixing

- Mother holds her breast to assist baby as needed, brings baby in close when his mouth is wide open. She may express drops of milk.
- Baby latches-on, takes all of nipple and about 2 cm (1 inch) of areola into mouth, then sucks, demonstrating recurrent burst-pause pattern.

4. Milk transfer

- Mother reports feeling any of the following: thirst, uterine cramps, increased lochia, breast ache or tingling, relaxation, sleepiness. Milk leaks from opposite breast.
- Baby swallows audibly; milk is observed in baby's mouth; baby may spit up milk when burping. Rapid "call up sucking" rate (2 sucks/second) changes to "nutritive sucking" rate of about 1 suck/second.

5. Ending

- Mother's breasts are comfortable; she lets baby suck until he is finished. After nursing, her breasts feel softer; she has no lumps, engorgement, or nipple soreness.
- Baby releases breast spontaneously, appears satiated. Baby does not root when stimulated. Baby's face, arms, and hands are relaxed; baby may fall asleep.

Mulford C (1992). The mother-baby assessment (MBA): An "Apgar score" for breastfeeding. *J Hum Lact*, 8:79–82. Reprinted with permission of Human Sciences Press, Inc., and the author.

The Infant Breastfeeding Assessment Tool (IBFAT) Method

Check the answer which best describes the baby's feeding behaviors at this feed.

1. When you picked baby up to feed was he/she			
(a) deeply asleep (eyes closed, no observable movement except breathing)	(b) drowsy	(c) quiet and alert	(d) crying

2. In order to get the baby to begin this feed, did you or the nurse have to			
(a) just place the baby on the breast as no effort was needed	(b) use mild stimulation such as unbundling, patting, or burping	(c) unbundle baby; sit baby back and forward; rub baby's body or limbs vigorously at the beginning and during the feeding	(d) baby could not be aroused
3	2	1	0

3. Rooting (definition: at touch of nipple to cheek, baby's head turns toward the nipple, the mouth opens, and baby attempts to fix mouth on the nipple). When the baby was placed beside the breast, he/she			
(a) rooted effectively at once	(b) needed some coaxing, prompting, or encouragement to root	(c) rooted poorly even with coaxing	(d) did not try to root
3	2	1	0

4. How long from placing baby at the breast does it take for the baby to latch-on and start to suck?			
(a) starts to feed at once (0–3 min)	(b) 3 to 10 minutes	(c) over 10 minutes	(d) did not feed
3	2	1	0

5. Which of the following phrases best describes the baby's feeding pattern at this feed?			
(a) baby did not suck	(b) sucked poorly; weak sucking; some sucking efforts for short periods	(c) sucked fairly well; sucked off and on, but needed encouragement	(d) sucked well throughout on one or both breasts
0	1	2	3

6. How do you feel about the way the baby fed at this feeding?			
(a) very pleased	(b) pleased	(c) fairly pleased	(d) not pleased

Source: Matthews MK (1988). Developing an instrument to assess infant breastfeeding behavior in the early neonatal period. *Midwifery*, 4(4),154–165. Reprinted with permission of Churchill Livingstone and the author.

Appendix G
WHO Growth Charts

Weight-for-Age Girls, Birth to 2 Years (Percentile)

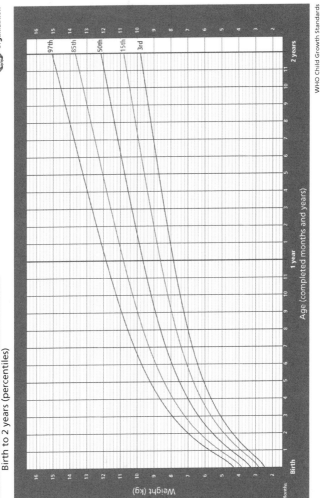

Weight-for-age BOYS
Birth to 2 years (percentiles)

Weight-for-Age Girls, Birth to 2 Years (Percentile)

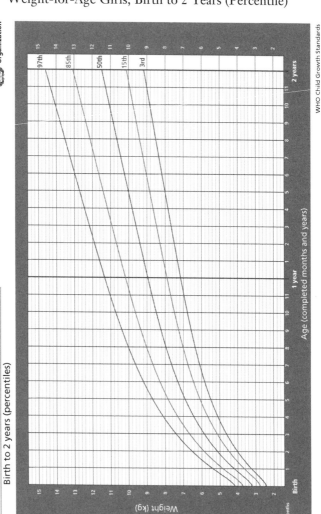

Appendix H
7 Percent Weight Loss—In Pounds and Ounces

For exact weight loss: Subtract current weight from birth weight and divide by birth weight.

Example: 7 lb 8 oz (120 oz) minus 7 lb 3 oz (115 oz) = 5 oz (birth weight minus current weight)

Divide: 5 divided by 120 = 4.2% weight loss

Source: International Lactation Consultant Association, 2007. Used with permission.

Weight	−7%	−10%	Weight	−7%	−10%
4.0	3.7	3.4	5.4	4.14	4.12
4.1	3.8	3.5	5.5	4.15	4.13
4.2	3.8	3.6	5.6	5.0	4.14
4.3	3.9	3.7	5.7	5.1	4.15
4.4	3.9	3.8	5.8	5.2	5.0
4.5	4.0	3.9	5.9	5.3	5.0
4.6	4.1	4.0	5.10	5.4	5.1
4.7	4.2	4.1	5.11	5.5	5.2
4.8	4.3	4.1	5.12	5.6	5.3
4.9	4.4	4.2	5.13	5.7	5.4
4.10	4.5	4.3	5.14	5.7	5.5
4.11	4.6	4.4	5.15	5.8	5.6
4.12	4.7	4.5	6.0	5.9	5.7
4.13	4.7	4.6	6.1	5.10	5.8
4.14	4.8	4.7	6.2	5.11	5.9
4.15	4.9	4.7	6.3	5.12	5.9
5.0	4.10	4.8	6.4	5.13	5.10
5.1	4.11	4.9	6.5	5.14	5.11
5.2	4.12	4.10	6.6	5.15	5.12
5.3	4.13	4.11	6.7	6.0	5.13

Weight	−7%	−10%	Weight	−7%	−10%
6.8	6.1	5.14	8.5	7.12	7.8
6.9	6.2	5.15	8.6	7.13	7.9
6.10	6.3	5.15	8.7	7.14	7.10
6.11	6.4	6.0	8.8	7.15	7.11
6.12	6.4	6.1	8.9	7.15	7.12
6.13	6.5	6.2	8.10	8.0	7.12
6.14	6.6	6.3	8.11	8.1	7.13
6.15	6.7	6.4	8.12	8.2	7.14
7.0	6.8	6.5	8.13	8.3	7.15
7.1	6.9	6.6	8.14	8.4	8.0
7.2	6.10	6.7	8.15	8.5	8.1
7.3	6.11	6.8	9.0	8.6	8.2
7.4	6.12	6.9	9.1	8.7	8.3
7.5	6.13	6.10	9.2	8.8	8.4
7.6	6.14	6.10	9.3	8.9	8.5
7.7	6.15	6.11	9.4	8.10	8.6
7.8	7.0	6.12	9.5	8.11	8.6
7.9	7.0	6.13	9.6	8.12	8.7
7.10	7.1	6.14	9.7	8.12	8.8
7.11	7.2	6.15	9.8	8.13	8.9
7.12	7.3	7.0	9.9	8.14	8.10
7.13	7.4	7.1	9.10	8.15	8.11
7.14	7.5	7.2	9.11	9.0	8.12
7.15	7.6	7.2	9.12	9.1	8.13
8.0	7.7	7.3	9.13	9.2	8.14
8.1	7.8	7.4	9.14	9.3	8.14
8.2	7.9	7.5	9.15	9.4	8.15
8.3	7.10	7.6	10.0	9.5	9.0
8.4	7.11	7.7			

7 and 10 Percent Weight Loss—In Grams

For exact weight loss: Subtract current weight from birth weight and divide by birth weight.

Example: 3402 grams minus 3260 grams = 142 (birth weight minus current weight)

Divide: 142 divided by 3402 = 4.2% weight loss

Source: International Lactation Consultant Association, 2007. Used with permission.

Weight	−0.07	−10%	Weight	−0.07	−10%
1814	1687	1633	2410	2241	2169
1843	1714	1659	2438	2267	2194
1871	1740	1684	2466	2294	2219
1899	1766	1709	2495	2320	2246
1928	1793	1735	2523	2347	2271
1965	1828	1769	2552	2373	2297
1984	1846	1786	2580	2399	2322
2013	1872	1812	2608	2426	2347
2041	1898	1837	2637	2452	2373
2070	1925	1863	2665	2478	2399
2098	1950	1888	2693	2505	2424
2126	1977	1913	2722	2531	2450
2155	2004	1940	2750	2557	2475
2183	2030	1965	2778	2584	2500
2211	2056	1990	2807	2610	2526
2240	2083	2016	2835	2637	2552
2268	2109	2041	2863	2663	2577
2296	2136	2066	2892	2689	2603
2325	2162	2093	2920	2716	2628
2353	2188	2118	2948	2742	2653
2381	2215	2143	2977	2768	2679

Weight	−0.07	−10%	Weight	−0.07	−10%
3005	2795	2705	3771	3507	3394
3033	2821	2730	3799	3533	3419
3062	2847	2756	3827	3559	3444
3090	2874	2781	3856	3586	3470
3119	2900	2807	3884	3612	3496
3147	2927	2832	3912	3638	3521
3175	2953	2858	3941	3665	3547
3204	2979	2884	3969	3691	3572
3232	3006	2909	3997	3718	3597
3260	3032	2934	4026	3744	3623
3289	3058	2960	4054	3770	3649
3317	3085	2985	4082	3797	3674
3345	3111	3011	4111	3823	3700
3374	3137	3037	4139	3849	3725
3402	3164	3062	4167	3876	3750
3430	3190	3087	4196	3902	3776
3459	3217	3113	4224	3928	3802
3487	3243	3138	4253	3955	3828
3515	3269	3164	4281	3981	3853
3544	3296	3190	4309	4008	3878
3572	3322	3215	4338	4034	3904
3600	3348	3240	4366	4060	3929
3629	3375	3266	4394	4087	3955
3657	3401	3291	4423	4113	3981
3686	3428	3317	4451	4139	4006
3714	3454	3343	4479	4166	4031
3742	3480	3368	4508	4192	4057

Appendix I
English—French—Spanish Glossary

English	French	Spanish
4 or more	Quatre ou plus	Cuatro o mas
8 to 12 times	Huit à douze fois	Ocho a doce veces
Allergy	Allergie	Alergia
Areola	Aréole	Areola
At least	Au moins	Por lo menos
Baby (your)	Votre bébé	Su bebé
Bottle	Bouteille	Biberón
Bottle-fed	Nourrir au biberon	Alimentado con biberón
Breast	Sein	El pecho el seno
Breast engorgement	Engorgement de sein	Congestión mamaria
Breast infection	Infection de sein	Infección mamaria
Breast massage	Massage de sein	Masaje del pecho
Breast pump	Pompe de sein	Sacaleches
Breastfeeding	Allaitement	Amamantar
Breastmilk	Lait de sein	Leche materna
Burp your baby	Roter votre bébé	Eructe su bebé
Colostrum (first milk)	La premier lait	La primera leche
Crying	Pleurer	Llanto
Doctor	Médecin	Doctor
Each day	Chaque jour	Cada día

English	French	Spanish
Enough	Assez	Suficiente
Exclusive breastfeeding	Par le sein exclusivement	Dar el pecho exclusivamente
Family	Famille	Familia
Father	Père	Padre
Feed your baby	Nourrir votre bébé	Déle pecho a su bebé
Feeding	Alimentation	Mamada
Flat nipple	Mamelon plats	Pezones planos
Food allergy	Allergie de nourriture	Alergia a las comidas
Gain weight	Gagner le poids	Ganar peso
Good afternoon	Bonjour	Buenas tardes
Good evening	Bonsoir	Buenas noches
Good morning	Bonne matin	Buenos días
Healthy	Sain	Saludable
Hormones	Hormones	Hormonas
Hospital	Hôpital	Hospital
How can I help you	Comment pouvoir je vous aide	Cómo puede yo le ayudo
How long	Comment longtemps	Cuánto tiempo
How many	Combien de	Cuántos
How much	Combien	Cuánto
How often	Combien de fois	Cada cuando
Husband	Mari	Esposo

English	French	Spanish
Inverted nipple	Mamelon inversé	Pezones invertidos
It's important	C'est important	Es importante
It's necessary	C'est nécessaire	Es necesario
Jaundice	Jaunisse	Ictericia
Lactation consultant	Consultant de lactation	Consultora en lactancia
Latch on (to)	S'accrocher	Agarrar
Letdown reflex	Réflexe de expulsion de lait	Reflejo de eyección de la leche
Meconium	Noircir et le poop épais	Popó negro y espeso
Medication	Médicaments	Medicina
Milk expression	Expression de lait	Extracción de la leche
Nipple	Mamelon	Pezón
Nipple shield	Protection de mamelon	Protectores flexibles para el pezón
Nurse (person)	Infirmière	Enfermera
Pacifier	Sucette	Chupete chupón
Please	S'il vous plaît	Por favor
Plugged duct	A bouché le conduit	Conducto obstruido
Premature	Prématuré	Prematuro
Problem	Problème	Problema
Reposition your baby better at the breast	Repositionner votre bébé mieux au sein	Reposicionar mejor el bebe al pecho
Return to work	Le retour pour travailler	Regresar al trabajo
Skin to skin	La peau pour écorcher	De piel a piel

English	French	Spanish
Sleep	Sommeil	Dormir
Sore nipple	Mamelon endolori	Pezones adoloridos
Spit up	Cracher en haut	Regugita
Suckle (to)	Allaiter	Amamantar mamar
Supplemental feeding	Alimentation additionelle	Alimentación suplementaria
Swallow (to)	Gorgée	Tragar
Thank you	Merci	Gracias
Wean	Sevrer	Destetar
You're welcome	De rien	De nada

Source: 2007 International Lactation Consultant Association. Used with permission.

INDEX

Note: Page numbers followed by *f* denote figures; those followed by *t* denote tables.

Scope of Practice for International Board Certified Lactation Consultants (IBCLCs)

International Board Certified Lactation Consultants (IBCLCs) have demonstrated specialized knowledge and clinical expertise in breastfeeding and human lactation and are certified by the International Board of Lactation Consultant Examiners (IBLCE).

This Scope of Practice encompasses the activities for which IBCLCs are educated and in which they are authorized to engage. The aim of this Scope of Practice is to protect the public by ensuring that all IBCLCs provide safe, competent and evidence-based care. As this is an international credential, this Scope of Practice is applicable in any country or setting where IBCLCs practice.

IBCLCs have the duty to uphold the standards of the IBCLC profession by:

- working within the framework defined by the IBLCE Code of Ethics, the Clinical Competencies for IBCLC Practice, and the International Lactation Consultant Association (ILCA) Standards of Practice for IBCLCs
- integrating knowledge and evidence when providing care for breastfeeding families from the disciplines defined in the IBLCE Exam Blueprint
- working within the legal framework of the respective geopolitical regions or settings
- maintaining knowledge and skills through regular continuing education

IBCLCs have the duty to protect, promote and support breastfeeding by:

- educating women, families, health professionals and the community about breastfeeding and human lactation
- facilitating the development of policies which protect, promote and support breastfeeding
- acting as an advocate for breastfeeding as the child-feeding norm
- providing holistic, evidence-based breastfeeding support and care, from preconception to weaning, for women and their families
- using principles of adult education when teaching clients, health care providers and others in the community
- complying with the International Code of Marketing of Breast-milk Substitutes and subsequent relevant World Health Assembly resolutions

IBCLCs have the duty to provide competent services for mothers and families by:

- performing comprehensive maternal, child and feeding assessments related to lactation

- developing and implementing an individualized feeding plan in consultation with the mother
- providing evidence-based information regarding a mother's use, during lactation, of medications (over-the-counter and prescription), alcohol, tobacco and street drugs, and their potential impact on milk production and child safety
- providing evidence-based information regarding complementary therapies during lactation and their impact on a mother's milk production and the effect on her child
- integrating cultural, psychosocial and nutritional aspects of breastfeeding
- providing support and encouragement to enable mothers to successfully meet their breastfeeding goals
- using effective counseling skills when interacting with clients and other health care providers
- using the principles of family-centred care while maintaining a collaborative, supportive relationship with clients

IBCLCs have the duty to report truthfully and fully to the mother and/or infant's primary health care provider and to the health care system by:

- recording all relevant information concerning care provided and, where appropriate, retaining records for the time specified by the local jurisdiction

IBCLCs have the duty to preserve client confidence by:

- respecting the privacy, dignity and confidentiality of mothers and families

IBCLCs have the duty to act with reasonable diligence by:

- assisting families with decisions regarding the feeding of children by providing information that is evidence-based and free of conflict of interest
- providing follow-up services as required
- making necessary referrals to other health care providers and community support resources when necessary
- functioning and contributing as a member of the health care team to deliver coordinated services to women and families
- working collaboratively and interdependently with other members of the health care team
- reporting to IBLCE if they have been found guilty of any offence under the criminal code of their country or jurisdiction in which they work or is sanctioned by another profession
- reporting to IBLCE any other IBCLC who is functioning outside this Scope of Practice